Situation, Field Perspective and Formation of Forms in Gestalt Therapy

This volume contains a collection of published and unpublished essays and conference lectures prepared by Jean-Marie Robine. Following the author in his line of thought, readers can learn how Robine has explored some of the topics most dear to him, in which his insights have become key contributions over the last ten years in the international Gestalt community.

Robine is one of the most prominent theorists on the contemporary gestalt therapy scene, and this book is a precious contribution to the gestalt therapy community not only for the contents it conveys, but as an example of a paradigmatic model of inquiry – of how to develop gestalt therapy theory and practice by drawing from various grounds and like-minded disciplines and channelling it into the practice of psychotherapy and stimulating new thought, without ever losing the rigour of our foundational epistemology. This new edition features five new chapters covering topics such as the concept of self, establishing a clinical approach to the "situation" in gestalt therapy and the therapeutic relationship.

Readers will be taken on a tour of Robine's unique perspectives in areas ranging from philosophical issues to social concerns, clinical insights to political perspectives, without ever losing focus of gestalt therapy. It will be of great value to therapists and students of gestalt therapy.

Jean-Marie Robine, PsyD, is a clinical psychologist and psychotherapist since 1967 and gestalt therapist since 1976. After more than 15 years as a psychologist, then director, in a public health service for children, adolescents and their families, he created in 1980 the Institut Français de Gestalt-thérapie (IFGT), the first Gestalt-therapy institute created in France which, to date, has trained hundreds or maybe thousands of gestalt therapists not only in France but also in Europe, Eastern Europe, Africa, USA and Latin America. He is a Fellow Member of the New York Institute for Gestalt Therapy. He is the author and editor of nine books on gestalt therapy and lives in the countryside, near Bordeaux, France.

The Gestalt Therapy Book Series

Istituto di Gestalt

www.gestaltitaly.com   HCC Italy

Series Editor **Margherita Spagnuolo Lobb**

The Istituto di Gestalt series of Gestalt therapy books emerges from the ground of a growing interest in theory, research and clinical practice in the Gestalt community. The members of the Scientific and Editorial Boards have been committed for many years to the process of supporting research and publications in our field: through this series we want to offer our colleagues internationally the richness of the current trends in Gestalt therapy theory and practice, underpinned by research. The goal of this series is to develop the original principles in hermeneutic terms: to articulate a relational perspective, namely a phenomenological, aesthetic, field-oriented approach to psychotherapy. It is also intended to help professions and to support a solid development and dialogue of Gestalt therapy with other psychotherapeutic methods.

The series includes original books specifically created for it, as well as translations of volumes originally published in other languages. We hope that our editorial effort will support the growth of the Gestalt therapy community; a dialogue with other modalities and disciplines; and new developments in research, clinics and other fields where Gestalt therapy theory can be applied (e.g., organizations, education, political and social critique and movements).

We would like to dedicate this Gestalt Therapy Book Series to all our mentors and colleagues who have sown fruitful seeds in our minds and hearts.

Coordinator
Stefania Benini

General Editor
Margherita Spagnuolo Lobb

Titles in the series:

For a full list of titles in this series, please visit www.routledge.com/Gestalt-Therapy/book-series/GESTHE and www.gestaltitaly.com

"Reminiscent of Laura Perls, Robine's approach to Gestalt therapy is philosophical and aesthetic, and his new publication is indeed 'true to form'. In his eloquent and deeply inspiring manner, Robine tempts readers to expand their horizons, explore unfamiliar places, and allow fresh impressions to linger. Whether revisiting familiar concepts or casting light on novel ones, Robine's focus on language is an invitation to rethink our convictions, deconstruct our conceptualizations, concentrate on contacting the Other, and embrace the situation we experience."

Nancy Amendt-Lyon, *Austrian Association for Gestalt Therapy and NYIGT*

Situation, Field Perspective and Formation of Forms in Gestalt Therapy

Social Change Begins with Two
Second Edition, Revised and Extended

Jean-Marie Robine

Translated from French by Claire Blatz,
Jean-Marie Robine, Karen Vincent Jones,
Olivier Winghart, Sonia Weyers

Routledge
Taylor & Francis Group
LONDON AND NEW YORK

Designed cover image: Courtesy of the painter Alain Bergeon
[www.alainbergeon.fr] © Alain Bergeon 2014

Second edition published in English 2026
by Routledge
4 Park Square, Milton Park, Abingdon, Oxon, OX14 4RN

and by Routledge
605 Third Avenue, New York, NY 10158

Routledge is an imprint of the Taylor & Francis Group, an informa business

© 2026 Jean-Marie Robine

The right of Jean-Marie Robine to be identified as author of this
work has been asserted in accordance with sections 77 and 78 of
the Copyright, Designs and Patents Act 1988.

Translated by Claire Blatz, Jean-Marie Robine, Karen Vincent Jones,
Olivier Winghart, Sonia Weyers.

First edition published in French by l'Exprimerie 2012
First edition published in English by Istituto di Gestalt HCC Italy 2015

British Library Cataloguing-in-Publication Data
A catalogue record for this book is available from the British Library

ISBN: 978-1-032-84949-2 (hbk)
ISBN: 978-1-032-84948-5 (pbk)
ISBN: 978-1-003-51576-0 (ebk)

DOI: 10.4324/9781003515760

Typeset in Times New Roman
by Apex CoVantage, LLC

Contents

Foreword to This Second Edition

The paradox that Carl Whitaker, the unclassifiable great therapist, liked to suggest can be extended to many other fields: "The best way to avoid psychotherapy is to have regular interviews with a therapist", he used to say. I will expand on this: the best way to avoid writing a book might be to publish essays on a regular basis. An essay is only a moment in the development of thought, a provisional formatting. It acknowledges the ephemeral nature of reflection, recognizing that the subject at hand cannot be defined here. Through the essay, we can attempt to rediscover the speaking speech/spoken speech dialectic put forward by Merleau-Ponty, and privilege the speaking word – even if it is written! – if we want to keep speech and thought alive.

These essays, grouped together under the title "Le changement social commence à deux" (Social Change Begins with Two), continue the process begun with my previous collection of essays, published under the title "S'apparaître à l'occasion d'un autre" (Self-appearing on the Occasion of Another). Should I have kept the same title for this new collection, simply adding "volume II" or even volume III or IV, since they were preceded by other texts? Is this not the same furrow I have been digging since I first encountered gestalt therapy some fifty years ago? That is also why this 2nd edition includes five new chapters compared with the previous edition.

Little by little, the paradigm shift suggested by the founders became clear to me. A hermeneutic dialogue began both with the founding text and with colleagues who were themselves groping in the same direction, sharing the same quest for coherence, extension and the unfolding of a text whose many parts continue to remain folded. And so, timidly in the eighties, more boldly in the nineties, what was awkwardly called the "field" (or "situation") perspective gradually took hold, as opposed to the no less awkwardly reductive perspective labelled "intrapsychic paradigm".

This revolution, which installed "contact" on the throne from which the "psyche" had reigned until then, has not finished opening up new avenues, since it has led me, and many others with me, to (attempt to) break with millennia-old habits, to see the world differently, to reframe many concepts and define new ones, and thus, in the domain that is mine-ours, to dare to consider allowing psychotherapy to develop outside its traditional roots. Some plants and trees not only draw on the deepest bowels of the earth for their growth, but have also added equally indispensable aerial roots for their vitality.

So I am not surprised that, when it came to naming this "new" psychotherapy, Laura Perls insisted – unsuccessfully – that the concept of *gestaltung* should be preferred rather than gestalt. That is because what we are interested in is movement, process, and not the fixed form that the concept of *gestalt* might imply. Hans Prinzhorn, the famous German psychiatrist who sparked our interest in what came to be known as *art brut* or *art of the insane*, elaborated his entire theory on the concept of *gestaltung* as early as the 1920s: "We seek the meaning of each formed form in the act of formation itself."

In this series of texts, which I did not intend to be a gestalt but rather a *gestaltung*, an act of forming forms, the reader is bound to notice the repetitions. To notice and perhaps to be annoyed. It is one of my ways of marking out my path. In other writings about psychotherapy, not included here, I like to look for support in aesthetics, and repetition as one of the major forms of contemporary creation – in music, dance, painting and poetry. In group situations, the words of one person are often linked to the words of another through a banal metaphor: "I'd like to bounce . . ." says the next speaker. Bouncing is another way of building on what has gone before. Perhaps it is to avoid repetition? In the art world, repetition has another name: *reprise*. In an article on the aesthetic approach to psychotherapy, I spoke of the aesthetics of reprise, darning being one of the translations for the French word *reprise*: both as in the theatre, when reprise evokes the possibility of breathing new life into a forgotten work, and in my own language, French, when darning-reprise referred to the sewing work carried out by generations before us, who "darned" socks, i.e. repaired them to put them back into circulation and prolong their existence.

Repetition is also a form of anaphora, a figure of speech that can express an obsession, but is also an insistence. I therefore suggest that readers try to overcome their possible irritation and consider my repetitions as an invitation. It is an invitation to visit a construction site, an invitation to accept my dissatisfaction with my previous thinking, an invitation to play with my trampoline and perhaps find pleasure in bouncing and bouncing . . .

To repeat the words of the philosopher Alain, who I am like: "Ideas, even the right ones, become false if we are content with them."

Foreword to the First Edition (2012)

On the Occasion of an Other, my previous work, was composed of a collection of essays and illustrations whose common element was the desire to deepen and refine the paradigm shift proposed by Gestalt therapy. In its founding text in 1951, in a form that is sometimes explicit and sometimes implicit, Gestalt therapy took the theory and practice of psychotherapy out of their solely intrapsychic reference in order to restructure them, within a field perspective, based on the concept of contact – which designates the internal movements of a field – and the formation of forms: in other words, a therapy of Gestalt.

The essays and conference lectures collected here are a continuation of my previous work. I have kept them in their original form; the reader will therefore come across a few repetitions since, in the independent context of each of these essays, it may have been useful or necessary to provide a foundation for the statements that followed.

Even though the following studies may seem to develop like a rhizome, they are drawn together by the title of the chapter that lends its name to the book: *Social Change Begins with Two*. Indeed, the relational dimension of psychotherapy will be a central theme here, as will the forms that it takes on and the references it puts into play. These studies were formulated against the backdrop of the threat made by certain obtuse politicians who claimed that the profession should be regulated. Now, "thanks" to them, professionals equipped with certain university degrees but without any specific training become *de facto* psychotherapists, while others, after being evaluated by the former group, may hope to be certified psychotherapists on the condition that they have an academic knowledge of psychopathology. While I certainly do not dispute the necessity of extensive psychopathological knowledge, the practice of psychotherapy cannot be limited to this qualification alone: the personal work carried out through in-depth personal psychotherapy, continuous supervision, relational expertise, a deontological commitment, and validation by one's peers – among other elements – constitute the fundamentals of the profession that was built upon these pillars, which together represented a training period that was six to eight times longer than that now required by the public authorities as a result of their pseudo-concern for safety!

Founding the profession on psychopathological knowledge alone engenders a practice that goes against what is proposed in this work. While a certain psychotherapy can exist under the medical model because it has its own indications, another is closer to a philosophical understanding of this specific work: an understanding that some will see as aesthetic, others as hermeneutic, but which will always have in common the fact that they are centred on the situation – on what takes place between a given psychotherapist and a particular patient.

The first part, entitled *How Situations Create Self*, contains different essays that approach certain fundamentals of Gestalt therapy. The first essay in particular, *The Self of the Situation*, reformulates and summarizes part of the theories I advanced in my previous work, which I hope will allow the reader to better understand the following essays, which build upon these foundations.

The second part, *How Situations Create Pathology*, addresses certain subjects related to psychopathology – that is to say, certain inflections of human experience that generate suffering. In particular, it contains two chapters on shame, a subject that is one of my main concerns and that I first began to study in 1990.

How Situations Create Forms is the title of the third part. In this section, the aesthetic paradigm is at the core of my reflection. *Form* is one of the possible – though insufficient – translations of the German concept of *Gestalt*. Gestalt therapy therefore means the therapy of the forms that each of us gives to our existence, our contacts, our relationships and our acts. Referring to aesthetics does not necessarily call upon the idea of beauty, but is based on *aesthesis* – what is felt – and the formation of forms.

Finally, the last section, *How Situations Create Encounters*, focuses on the processes, events and modalities – and their consequences – of what is woven between the therapist and the patient, and what is commonly referred to as "the therapeutic relationship". Here we are far from the myth of neutrality that for a long time hovered over the profession and whose shadow is still felt today! The last chapter, "What I believe and what I believe that I believe", could be considered a conclusion, if we wanted to accord it this provisional role. Part of my credo is that certain convictions must be able to change over the years, and after 57 years practising psychotherapy and 47 years gestalt therapy, I certainly think I have fewer certitudes than I did at the outset.

Jean-Marie Robine

Acknowledgements

I'd like to thank everyone who has helped and supported me over the years, both colleagues and students. Their comments, questions, invitations and challenges have always been what has sparked my research and my reflections.

First of all, Brigitte Lapeyronnie-Robine, my partner and most dedicated reader, ever attentive and supportive with a critical eye for detail.

My trainer-colleagues at the Institut Français de Gestalt-thérapie (French Institute for Gestalt Therapy): Brigitte again, as well as Anne Chrétien[†], Christiane Garrivet, Ximo Tarrega, Pierre-Yves Goriaux, Dominique Michel, Elvira Dueñas, Françoise Dero, Jean-Pierre Garrivet, and the trainers who often work in association with our Institute: André Lamy, Nicole de Schrevel, Jacques Blaize, Marie Petit[†], Patrick Colin, Edith Blanquet, Nadine Gardahaut . . .

And all my foreign colleagues who have given me the pleasure of being part of their reflections and/or the training they provide, particularly Michael V. Miller, Daniel Bloom, Ruella Frank, Myriam Muñoz Polit[†], Carmen Vázquez Bandín, Mônica Botelho Alvim, Marcos and Rosane Müller-Granzotto, Selma Ciornai, Myriam Sas de Guiter, Marta Slemenson, Claudia Tovora, Margherita Spagnuolo Lobb, Gianni Francesetti, Mariano Pizzimenti, Tomaž Flajs, Rudi Kotnik, Natacha Kedrova, Daniel Khlomov, Elena Mazur, Yuri Shevcenko, Anna Bychkova, Inna Didkovskaya, Albina Martynova, Olya Yvtushenko, Alexandre Mokhovikov[†], Elena Petrova, Serguey Kondurov . . .

And to revise and extend this second edition, I want to specifically thank the editorial board of this collection led by Margherita Spagnuolo Lobb. With her, Stefania Benini, Annette Hillers-Chen, Jay Tropianskaia, Andy Williams and Jelena Zeleskov Djoric joined their advice, suggestions and support which were priceless!

Preface of the First American-English Edition, 2012

Gianni Francesetti

Psychiatrist, Gestalt therapist
President of European Association for Gestalt Therapy

Social Change Begins with Two is a collection of published and unpublished essays and conference lectures prepared by Jean-Marie Robine over the last ten years. Its release is a unique opportunity to be taken on a tour of his thought over the decade and its developments in areas ranging from philosophical issues to social concerns, clinical insights to political perspectives, without ever losing focus of Gestalt therapy, the thread unifying the collection. Following the author in his line of thought, readers can learn how Jean-Marie has explored some of the topics most dear to him, in which his insights have become key contributions over the last ten years to debate in the international Gestalt community. Robine is one of the most prominent theorists on the contemporary Gestalt therapy scene. For years he has developed a discourse that is firmly rooted in the epistemology of the paradigm, bringing forth new, stimulating figures that are a creative inspiration for his students and readers.

These contributions represent a continuous dialogue between the theoretical roots of Gestalt therapy and the latest developments in the field. A primary characteristic of these essays is the way they combine theoretical rigour and epistemological consistency with an openness towards the growing edge of contemporary Gestalt therapy. Secondly, they build bridges and connections with a number of the disciplines that constantly inform Gestalt therapy theory and practice. One example, which I believe is a specific element of Jean-Marie Robine's thought and which I appreciate very much for my affinity with it, is his ability to draw from Gestalt psychology and from phenomenology to develop and shed new light on theory. With regard to phenomenology in particular, he builds on the rich tradition of phenomenological psychiatry, which in France enjoyed extraordinary growth in the twentieth century and which the author is versed in perfectly.

His is a dialogue, therefore, that endlessly plays with the underpinnings of Gestalt therapy, without ever losing strict sight of the foundation text by Perls, Hefferline and Goodman, without which any development would be cut off from its roots and unable to grow. The experience of this dialogue leaves readers with a vision that is broader, a horizon that is vaster and in constant motion, never crystallized within the immobilizing constraints of a system. It supports Gestalt therapy in practice by uniting creativity with consistency, theoretical vision with the contextual specificity of every encounter and philosophical exploration with the needs of patients and society today.

I would also like to underscore some of the points that, in my view, render Robine's perspective so fundamental and so stimulating for contemporary Gestalt therapists, and I shall do so by highlighting some of the issues that readers will come across in this book.

To begin with, the epistemology of every subject explored by the author can never be reduced to the individual. A look at the individual is never sufficient to understand the human being. It is the field – or the situation or the relationship – that needs to be taken as the minimum unit and starting point for any anthropological or therapeutic consideration of human beings. Such solicitude permeates the book in both its theoretical elements and practical sides, warning readers of how easy it is to slip into an individualistic approach to therapy that stands in contrast with our perspective. In this regard, the book features some wonderful passages on the situational self, on shame, on emotions as phenomena of the field and on the clinical and social implications of a radically relational perspective.

A second aspect I believe to be very important is the concept of the emergence of the self and the individual from the "vague and confused" of the ground through a process of progressive differentiation. Jean-Marie focuses on this aspect in various ways, by pausing, for instance, on an analysis of forecontact and enriching the perspective through the lens of Gestalt psychology and phenomenology. By focusing on this moment of experience he identifies an important implication for therapy when he stresses the need to avoid precociously defining what happens at the contact boundary, but rather to accompany the emergence of the figure by fostering co-creation, a process that is interrupted if the therapist is unable to tolerate the uncertainty and fragility that we inevitably encounter at the dawning of the experience. A lack of care at this stage risks not only being ineffective but can be harmful for the patient as it does not let his/her intentionality emerge at the contact boundary and can invalidate the experience by introducing feelings of shame, invasion or confusion, if the boundaries are not sufficiently set. This focus on shaping experience from a moment of indifferentiation also opens up a more original and productive understanding of psychotic experiences (in this regard see the chapter on psychosis by Francesetti and Spagnuolo Lobb in Francesetti, Gecele, Roubal (Eds.) *Gestalt Therapy in Clinical Practice*, 2013).

Another issue the author explores in a very original way is that of psychopathology. The issue emerges in various chapters, with a viewpoint of psychopathology that draws critically from psychiatric traditions, dialogues with contemporary views and returns to the epistemology of Gestalt therapy, offering readers a panorama of the field that is never simplistic and always true to its inherent complexity.

Finally, there is the topic of society and politics, which is reflected in the title of the book. Remaining faithful to the social mission that Gestalt therapy has had ever since its beginnings, in various passages Robine establishes the interconnection between society and psychotherapy, highlighting how the former can give rise to social change and how the latter can be a source of suffering but also a space for "healing". In this way the role of the psychotherapist is seen to be both in and out of the therapeutical room, one that is rooted in society at large but that strives to give meaning to his/her work in the intimacy of therapy. Such an understanding helps remediate the reductionism that sees the psyche reduced to a purely intimate, internal phenomenon, when instead it is a vibration at the contact boundary, a place of inspiration and social encounter.

This book is a precious contribution to the Gestalt therapy community not only for the contents it conveys, but as an example of a paradigmatic model of inquiry – of how to develop Gestalt therapy theory and practice by drawing from various grounds and like-minded disciplines and channelling it all into the practice of psychotherapy and stimulating new thought, without ever losing the rigour of our foundational epistemology. The deliberate non-systematicity of the paths presented leaves matters open rather than closing them, encouraging readers to explore the outlines and suggestions provided by the author, in what is a rather effective way of not precociously closing the horizons that these pages throw open.

A book that every Gestalt therapist should read to refresh their critical understanding of our roots in dialogue with the contemporary world. A journey back to the roots of our model, to emerge afresh with a renewed sense of awareness and new words.

How Situations Create Self

Chapter 1

The Self of the Situation

Sixty years ago, with *Gestalt Therapy* Perls and Goodman introduced an essential turning point that propelled them into the very heart of contemporary reflection: they displaced the self, delocalized it and situated it in time. In the "modern", largely solipsistic approach, the individual self was recognized as the only reality, with the psyche as one of its main variations. Based on the simplest primary reality, i.e. that all human functions involve contact with the environment, Perls and Goodman structured a fundamentally innovative praxis and idea, directly related to this natural understanding of human nature.

At the time, the concept of "self" had barely entered the psychoanalytic and psychotherapeutic vocabulary, not yet having experienced the glory days to which authors like Winnicott and Kohut would later introduce it. When it was used, it was often reduced to partial aspects and became an entity that was more or less endowed with stability. This is often still the case today. In gestalt therapy, what we call "self" only exists when and where there is contact. According to this understanding, the self is not alleged to have previously existed and then to reveal, manifest and express itself through contact, but rather it *is* contact. The self is folding and unfolding: movement. It is the implementation of creative adjustments that take place at the organism/environment contact boundary. In a field defined as "an organism and its environment", the self-function refers to the internal movements of this field: movements of integration and differentiation, unification and individuation, action and transformation . . . To be able to grow and develop, the organism must encounter what is new, different, and not itself; it gives it shape – that is to say, it constructs a gestalt – and as part of the operation of contact that it thereby carries out, driven by the excitement that accompanies this "formation of form", it is returned to this continued individuation: this self/world differentiation which is repeated unceasingly. This process is called self. "The self is only a small factor in the total organism/environment interaction, but it plays the crucial role of developing and creating meanings that enable us to grow."

This relocation of the self and its repositioning as a field phenomenon may elicit a great deal of surprise, since it pre-empted the work of many philosophers, sociologists and essayists of the second half of the twentieth century. However, throughout the pages of *Gestalt Therapy*, the attentive reader will not fail to

DOI: 10.4324/9781003515760-2

perceive some oscillations between a traditional concept of a self-entity (some-times called a "self-object" by certain later authors) and the innovative concept that they introduced, and with it a new paradigm that was later developed – often less radically – by certain authors of postmodernism, social constructionism and intersubjective psychoanalysis, as well as other identity theorists.

Reaffirming the innovative nature of their work, the authors do not seek to base their approach on any type of metapsychology, although they often allow the reader to perceive the admiration – not without criticism – they had for Freud. They prefer to draw on anthropology, a conception of man-in-the-world, and – perhaps most importantly – the therapeutic situation itself. While they bor-row certain concepts from psychoanalysis, they redefine them by opening them up to the situational field perspective. For example, the Freudian "id", as the pri-mary reservoir of instinctual energy, makes way for the "id of the situation", per-fectly confirming the paradigm shift that has taken place. Psychotherapy is thus no longer defined as an expert's implementation of acquired knowledge that is expressed through interpretations or other specialist acts; it is first and foremost "situation": a contact situation, here and now, "reality" as well as a metaphor or metonymy of the past, future and elsewhere. If humans create and are created by situations, psychotherapy can act as a sort of laboratory; developing an aware-ness of contacts, its interruptions and its inflections will confirm gestalt therapy's method as an application of phenomenology to the clinical realm and, dare we say, as a veritable analysis of *Dasein*.

Gestalt Therapy opens with the following words, inspired by the Aristote-lian tradition: "Experience occurs at the boundary between the organism and its environment." The book ends with: "In an experience rich in contact, the 'I' [. . .] identifies with the developing self [. . .] and, at the moment of accom-plishment, disappears from the path." In the span of a few dozen pages, we have crossed the gulf separating Aristotle from the philosophy of Tao, two approaches that were highly valued by the authors. Between the two, Kant and Freud, William James and Kurt Lewin, Wertheimer and Croce, Otto Rank and Paul Fed-ern, Martin Buber, Proust and many others are drawn upon to enrich a reflection which, as Perls suggests, cannot be massively introjected without dental aggres-sion, without creation on the part of the reader, without incarnation in one's own experience.

The work bequeathed by gestalt therapy's founders requires an extensive amount of complementary development. Today, the trails they blazed some sixty years ago are far from having become high traffic roads. This task falls to those who iden-tify as their successors; it is indeed a daunting task if they are not to reduce the founders' visionary advances to a simplistic set of devices, as has unfortunately sometimes been the case over the past few decades. Throughout this essay, I wish to draw some of their initial proposals further into the foreground, or even to radi-calize them, with the hopes of preserving the spirit that presided over the shaping of their theories.

Self as Unfolding

The self is not *only* an entity, and therefore not only refers to the id-entity. Certainly one of the major difficulties that we encounter in understanding gestalt therapy's theory of self, and consequently its widespread clinical use, lies in the different readings of our conception of the "self". We are subject to a cultural tendency that urges us to draw the self toward the subject, toward the person, and thus to reify it, to assign it contours, just as we find it difficult not to think of ourselves with me/not-me contours . . . One of the major challenges of twentieth-century thought concerning these topics is the superposition of the concept of self – or of subject – with that of person or individual. If we want to understand the work of Goodman (and that of many thinkers of the second half of the last century), it seems necessary to differentiate between these concepts and not to conflate "self" and "person", or "subject" and "individual."

"Self" refers to an operation of turning toward the origin of the action. It is a reflexive operation by which the actor is specified, limited and defined. This operation presupposes integration into a field to achieve ongoing differentiation. It is individuation, not the individual. It is Montaigne's "I do not paint the being; I paint the passage". *Self* thus designates the reflexive operation that constitutes this self/world differentiation, as well as (but only as a consequence of this primary designation) the result of this operation.

This "result" that we call "self" also indicates our difference from the other. It is not my intention here to present a selection of quotes from Perls and Goodman to highlight how our founding text constantly oscillates between these two conceptions of the self: one that suggests it is an entity versus one that suggests it is an operator; one that suggests it is a body full of needs and desires versus one that emphasizes the need for the unceasing creation of meanings; one that defines contact-with-the-world as "a going toward and taking from" versus one that evokes it in terms of creative adjustment and the construction/destruction of gestalts. We recognize a certain tension, which is not always dialectical, between the proposals made by Perls and those made by Goodman.

But what matters to me here is clarifying the conception of the self that is used in psychotherapy.

If we define psychotherapy as:

- an act of intervention on psychological contents,
- an expert act in personality organization,
- the action of a changer in favour of an other who is changing/a changed future,
- the reduction of a pathology – and of the associated suffering – with reference to an extrinsic norm and a definition of what is healthy/unhealthy . . .

. . . we will doubtless need to rely on a conception of the self that theorizes it as an entity, and we can easily understand how tempting it is to turn to one of the theories that make proposals on the internal organization of the individual, its manifestations and structures, its "object relations" or other so-called "internal" structures.

But if we define psychotherapy as a meeting that allows for an "appearing", "appearing in the openness of a situation" or, as I like to say it, "appearing on the occasion of an other", priority will be placed on this reflexivity of the self, this movement of the field that, based on this "between", supports continuous individuation.

The process of revelation thus seeks "to understand the individual based on individuation, rather than individuation based on the individual" (Simondon, 1964). It is the operation of taking shape that defines the being; a being before individuation is a field rich with potential that can only be by becoming: that is to say, by individuating. This is what the therapist assists in doing: he or she guides the being in its genesis.

Substantialist tradition encourages us to persist in a misunderstanding of "the relationship", which is understood as a relation between terms which exist prior to the act of linking them together. If we follow Simondon in his proposals, which invert the traditional viewpoint, the study of individuation is the substance (which here could refer to the individual as the fixture of a process) "[a]n extreme case of the relationship: that of the inconsistency of the relationship" (Simondon, 1964). It suggests that only a theory that envisages a being through the multitude of operations in which this being individuates will be able to transform the approach to the relationship: "the being appears as what becomes by connecting."

Thus the individual *consists* of connections. And this "consists" should be understood on two levels:

- the individual is nothing but relationships: the operations of individuation that each of us renews and which create each of us by establishing the individual as a link between the varied levels of his or her experience,
- and it is also the relationship that gives consistency to a being: that is to say, his or her reality.

The individual is both what acts in the relationship and what results from it. Any change in an individual's relation to others is also a change in its "internal" characteristics. Moreover, any difference between "internal" and "external" is only a relative distinction, since what is outside the individual can get inside, just as what is inside can get out. This is of course the movement that governs growth. One of Goodman's fundamental intuitions resides in this premise: we do not understand what an individual's reality may *consist* of until we understand the importance of that individual's relationship with his or her environment, since the individual considered in isolation is an incomplete reality, and only the relational act can enable contact operations to be converted into structure, and structure into contact operations.

Self in Situation/of Situation

As I see it, psychotherapy is thus faced with the choice between either:

- relying on the model of a one-person psychology, such as that of classical psychoanalysis, which establishes the therapist in a certain type of presence and function, or
- being part of a two-person psychology, a model launched by Ferenczi and developed by Balint, Winnicott and many others, and the therapist will no longer be a stranger to the field of experience.

Our founding authors provided us with a work that oscillates between these two poles:

The influence of Perls and his conception of contact as a "going toward and taking from" would bring us closer to "object seeking", as Fairbairn, for example, puts it, which hardly involves any fundamental epistemological break with the theory of instinct developed by Freud.

Goodman's influence, on the other hand, is felt through his approach which considers contact as creative adjustment, as the construction of the meaning of experience in an organism/environment field.

The point at which our two authors converge is in the importance they attach to the field and its immediate consequence: a specific theory of the self. But given their specific premises, in Perls' vision the field and the self are often reified, while Goodman approaches the field and the self more as processes undergoing ongoing development.

The Lewinian approach suggested by Perls and Goodman is far from homogeneous. Under this approach, the field is seen as a "force field" that exerts itself on a given subject. The use of the reference to the magnetic field is an interesting metaphor when called upon in one-person psychology; it becomes more dangerous in psychology involving two or more people, since it is difficult to avoid reifying the interpersonal or group-level "field".

The reference to the field, which Perls and Goodman use as a foundation, is much closer to a phenomenological understanding, which involves the field of awareness or that of experience. From this perspective, which could be described as subjective or experiential, the field would constitute this experienced "space" of perceptions, actions, feelings and meanings of a given individual.

When referring to contact and other field phenomena, Perls and Goodman periodically introduced the distinction between "in the field" and "of the field". Place the subject, the body, the contact, etc. as events *of* the field and not *in* the field clarifies the matter by opposing the two major uses of the concept of field: one that results in reification and the other that maintains the field in flux.

Nevertheless, we should note that although Perls and Goodman place the issue of the field at the centre of the theoretical system they develop, they rarely mention it directly. However, careful study reveals that they make very frequent use of the concept of *situation*, which I will briefly focus on since I believe it represents a substantial opportunity for refining and clarifying the perspective that it introduces.

Every therapeutic system is first and foremost a certain type of situation. Being aware of how the situation has an impact on us is also a way of better understanding how we have been affected by certain situations throughout our personal history. Being aware of how we can be creators or co-creators of situations in the here and now is also a way of restoring or enhancing our abilities to creatively adjust.

The starting point of my question on "the situation", and of the surprises that ensued, is found in a "little" phrase of Perls and Goodman in which they mention the "id of the situation," without much further development! (Once again, they are not talking about the id *in* a situation but rather the id *of* the situation!) It is up to us to try to resolve or understand this surprising proposal, which leads us far off the beaten tracks pioneered by Groddeck or Freud, far from the theory of drives and of these so-called inner forces that drive us. I then discovered that on many occasions, our authors relied heavily on the concept of situation; for example, one of the defining characteristics of the self is being "engaged in the situation", neurosis is described as "a chronic, low-intensity emergency situation", psychotherapy itself is primarily and most frequently described in terms of situation, such as in these lines, which are found in the general introduction:

> The therapeutic *situation* is more than a statistical event of doctor plus a patient. [. . .] Neither the full understanding of the organismic functions nor the best knowledge about the environment (society, etc.) covers the total *situation*. Only the interplay of organism and environment constitutes the psychological *situation*, not the organism and environment taken separately. [. . .]
>
> [W]e change our outlook toward the therapeutic *situation* [. . .] [T]he clinical becomes an experimental *situation* . . .
>
> (Perls, Hefferline & Goodman, 1951, pp. xi–xii; emphasis my own)

I have often been surprised to note that the vast majority of gestalt therapists eagerly develop their skills towards a better understanding of "organismic functions" (biology, studies on the brain and other functions explored by neuroscience, theories of the psyche, etc.) and that far fewer of them sought "the best knowledge about the environment (society, etc.)" through sociology, ecology, anthropology, etc. While all these approaches have their merits, our authors explicitly state in the quote above that we should not stop at what they call "abstractions" elsewhere (to refer to both the organism and the environment, considered in isolation), and that we should instead explore further at the level of "the situation".

This concept of situation is so commonly used, it rarely appears as such in the discussion. It is a backdrop that is taken for granted, implicit and rarely questioned. However, over the past several decades various researchers, especially those surrounding and following Erving Goffman and the Chicago School (Goffman, 1964), have placed the concept of situation at the heart of their work. Furthermore, the interest in this approach can without a doubt be traced back to John

Dewey. It is also worth remembering that Dewey had a significant impact on Goodman's intellectual development. Therefore, as a side note, the fundamental distinction between "in the field" and "of the field" mentioned above, which Goodman introduced, comes straight from Dewey, who was fond of specifying that an organism does not live *in* an environment, but "*by means of* an environment" (Dewey, 1933).

When Perls and Goodman, addressing the characteristics of the self, describe it as "engaged in the situation", they specify: "[By this] we mean that there is no sense of oneself or of other things other than one's experience of the situation" (Perls, Hefferline and Goodman, 1951, 10, *4*). I am made by the situation just as much as I participate with the other in creating the situation. Before a gestalt even begins to be take effect in the therapy session, the situation has already started being created and will serve as a backdrop to the figures to come. Whatever the situation may be, the self either unfolds or doesn't in connection with this situation. If we accept the concept of a self as a moving function of the field, which is mobilized when and because a creative adjustment is at work, we are particularly susceptible to developing conditions favourable to actualizing or restoring the self. The self allows routines, secondary physiology and systems of habits to carry out minimal adjustments; neurosis, defined as the loss of function of the self, may thus be regarded as a denial of the situation. The neurotic individual acts as though the novelty of the situation here and now did not exist: as if this situation could be reduced to a few of its constituents, fixed once and for all in the form of patterns of thought, feeling and action.

Let us return to the definition of neurosis as "a situation of chronic low-grade emergency" and to the conclusions that Perls and Goodman draw from it with regard to therapy. Placed in a new situation of imbalance, danger, threat or survival, which the authors of *Gestalt Therapy* refer to by the generic term "emergency", the organism develops a comprehensive, adapted response: comprehensive because it involves perceptions, proprioceptions, representations and thought, motor activity, etc.; adapted because the possibility at the contact boundary that actualizes itself through this process allows the event to be spontaneously, creatively dealt with. Orientation and manipulation capabilities in the field unfold to their fullest extent and resist the disruption of the field.

But through repetition and the failure to restore balance or find "refuge in repression or hallucination", a chronicity of the imbalance and the adaptive gestalt will take place at a low intensity. The tension will thus be twofold: danger AND frustration, which mutually provoke each other to the point of neurosis. This is what Perls and Goodman call "a situation of chronic low-grade emergency", which they offer as one of the definitions of neurosis. In this situation, the experience at the contact boundary tends to simplify the field by involving two emergency functions: deliberate repression and unintentional hyperactivity:

If the neurotic state is the response to a non-existent chronic low-grade emergency, with medium tonus and dull and fixed alertness instead of either relaxation or galvanic tone and sharp flexible alertness, then the aim is to concentrate on an existing high-grade emergency with which the patient can actually cope and thereby grow.

(Perls, Hefferline & Goodman, 1951, p. 288)

Psychotherapy is thereby conceived of as an opposing situation of emergency, which borrows a number of parameters from the chronic emergency situation but which – in this new, safe, experimental context – deprives the patient of his or her obsolete answers to encourage the creation of new solutions that are adjusted to the novelty of the situation. We must "concentrate on the structure of the actual situation as the task of creative adjustment; to try for an altogether new synthesis and make this the chief point of the session" (Perls, Hefferline and Goodman, 1951, 4, *11*). At the risk of belabouring the point, let us recall that this ability is what gestalt therapy calls "self". The work of restoring the self thus appears much more related to a rootedness in the situation than to one person's expertise concerning the psyche of the other.

Consideration of the situation, "the id of the situation", therefore takes place from the very first moments of each therapeutic encounter and is an integral part of what we call "pre-contact". But pre-contact should not only be considered as a *moment* in the sequence of contact; it is also a modality of this sequence. Some-times, even during later developmental stages of the gestalt, we are led to "return" to the situation, to make it more precise and more explicit, and thus help to clarify and intensify the figure/ground relation. Development theorists have repeatedly emphasized that each new phase does not replace the previous one, but instead is added to it, and that the contents of each phase continue to be developed, even at later stages. During an interview a few years ago (Robine, 1992), Erv Polster told me that probably the most important thing he had learned from Paul Goodman was to consider the adult state as a "plus" to childhood and not a "then" . . . This logic of "at the same time as", as opposed to "instead of", actually runs throughout *Gestalt Therapy*. Development, which is built over the years according to these modalities, is present in the construction of a gestalt, which occurs over a shorter period of time during the therapy session. The situation, if it can be considered as a sort of base for the therapeutic encounter, is developed throughout each session. It is often useful to clarify its constituents as they evolve, since this situation creates us at the same time as we create it.

When a patient sits across from me and tells me he is anxious, I can choose to take his words not only as words spoken *in* a certain situation, but also as words *of* the situation, *as if* these words belonged to an undifferentiated field that will need be to clarified rather than to the individual who uttered them. The classical individualist position would focus, as I did for years, on *the patient's* anxiety: how he feels this anxiety, where it comes from, what it reminds him of, through which projections it may be organized, etc. This position leads the therapist to believe that he or she is gaining ever more detailed knowledge of the patient. However, although this position may seem just as "natural" as it is usual, it is only a "choice" that stems from a prejudice.

Another choice, associated with another prejudice, lets me regard this anxiety as belonging "first" to the situation. Perhaps this anxiety is his response to the view he has of me? Perhaps I make him anxious? Perhaps I make him anxious in reaction to the view I have of him, or of our encounter? Perhaps "his" anxiety is only my own? Or is it only the atmosphere that is immediately created between us?

My choice to start with the situation is in no way based on any truth: it is not a methodological choice, based on a theoretical choice. What I usually call "myself" can often be approached as a premature differentiation of the field. "Experience is prior to the 'organism' and the 'environment', which are abstractions from experience" (Goodman, 1972, p. 7). Progressive, continuous differentiation; round trips back and forth between integration and individuation; the consequent destabilization of the rigid system of self-representations (this is me/this isn't me), etc. are at the heart of therapeutic work and the construction of the self through reflexivity.

This position diverges somewhat from the dialogical position, although many of the proposals it develops are not so different. While the dialogical perspective takes into account the issue of the field, I find that it functions as if two distinct individuals had already been clearly identified: two subjects who meet and transform their experience. I consider this more an epistemology "in the field" than "of the field": two people who are already individuated, rather than the progressive individuation of two people. Temporalization is not approached in the same way, despite the fact that, in the situational perspective that I recommend, the dialogical component is readily implemented. We cannot help but be reminded of one of the main functions of speech highlighted by many theorists: speaking is an attempt to fill this self/ other gap, to overcome the original separation and grasp at the fleeting illusion of achieving this for a few moments . . . but it also means being doomed to fail at this attempt, to endlessly renew this futile attempt like a sort of Sisyphus, rolling his verbal boulder up the mountain only to see it topple back down the other side.

During this process of individuation, there are times when *I* am I and you are *you* and where we can meet, certainly, but there are also times when I am *you* and you are *I*, others where there is only a *one*, others where there is a *we*, albeit illusory, and still others where I have no idea who I am or who you are!

These movements *of* the field (or *of* the situation), which allow this reflexivity toward one and the other as distinctive subjects, are the movements of contact. I have often had occasion to emphasize that gestalt therapy is much more of a verb culture than a noun culture, a culture more of the act than the entity. Following this logic, when I listen to a patient, including his retelling of anecdotes or dreams, I focus on the verbs that are used, which may be considered clues about the movements of the situation. If he tells me, for example, that in his dream he dropped his book, rather than considering this an "insignificant" detail, I could focus on this "dropping" or "letting go" and explore its possible meanings: an unconscious desire to give up therapy? Fear that I'll abandon him? And so on.

This focus on the situation in an attempt to identify its components has also led me to be more sensitive to what is there, and to focus more on it than on what is not there. Premature attention paid to what is not there contains an implicit "should be there" which is almost inevitable and generates shame. Noting that the patient is looking insistently at the painting hanging on the wall behind me is not quite the same as noting that he is not looking at me. Noting that he has adopted a constricted breathing pattern is not the same as noting that he is hardly breathing. Noting that he expresses himself evenly is not the same thing as stressing that he doesn't let his emotions show . . .

The gestalt therapist, who is familiar with approaching all human activities (thinking, acting, talking, reacting emotionally, exploring the environment, etc.) as contact-boundary phenomena – i.e. as modes of contact – can easily consider these activities as "situated activities".

> Situations do not cause our actions, but they do not represent a simple background against which we realize our intentions, either. We only perceive a situation according to our aptitudes and our current preparedness to act.
>
> (Joas, 1992)

I will relate one of my favourite examples. During our first or second interview together, a woman in her sixties told me about her life of abundance and her weariness faced with the numerous intrusions of her children and grandchildren, who invaded her life and devoured it. It was a beautiful late afternoon in summertime and a particularly intense ray of sunlight had hit her face and was blinding her but without her seeming to notice that it was bothering her. ("Seen but unnoticed", as situation theorists like to say.) Simply moving her chair a few inches to one side was enough to avoid this solar intrusion that was making her grimace in discomfort. But "we only perceive a situation according to our aptitudes and our current preparedness to act", as Joas put it, and clearly the absence of provisions to act prevented her from perceiving the situation . . . Working with her on her family relationships or her difficulty setting boundaries and limits would probably be quite ineffective until she was more aware of her direct contact with the situation than what she demonstrated *in situ*.

The gestalt therapist works on the process of constructing figures ("the therapy – or analysis – of the gestalt", Perls, Hefferline and Goodman, 1951, I, 7). But it is not so much the figure itself that holds our attention as the relationship that the figure has with the ground that constitutes it and supports it. A figure in isolation has no meaning. Marcel Duchamp, by taking a urinal out of the ordinary context of a bathroom and displaying it on a pedestal in a sculpture museum, made a striking demonstration: he reimagined the situation, "situating" the act and the object differently. This fundamental act is a crucial starting point for the gestalt therapist and also draws our attention to the specificity of the "here" in the here and now of each encounter.

In the Situation, Exposing Intentionality

When one person sits across from another, something happens: they create a situation and at the same time they are created by the situation. According to a traditional way of thinking, one's speech, behaviour, expression and actions are generally approached and understood as singular experiences specific to a given individual. The meaning of what this person shows, and what he or she is, is considered the product of his or her personal history, development, social conditions, physiology, etc. Understanding meaning in this way is a choice that fits within a single-person psychology: that is to say, a solipsistic or intrapsychic epistemology.

This choice has its validity and, indeed, everything – every event that is to come – can validate this way of thinking.

We may also have other assumptions, other choices, related to a field perspective. Let us assume that in such a situation, speech, behaviour, expression, actions, emotions and feelings are immediately and implicitly related to the field – to the organization/environment field: in other words, to what is experienced as "me" and what is experienced as "not-me", notably including the other. The individualistic perspective more readily connects the majority of experience to the individual who experiences it – the actor, which represents only a small part of the whole field.

Some may object that in many cases, particularly towards the beginning of therapy, the client hardly seems aware of the therapist's presence. To put it in a somewhat less schematic way, the patient seems driven by an urgent need to talk, not by the need to talk *to*, or *someone* to talk to, let alone the need to talk to *me* . . .

Once again, let us consider that this is one of the possible ways of understanding the situation, one which is so embedded in our habits and in the patient's habits and ways of thinking, it is practically a belief.

Faced with this belief, I made the choice to oppose a different *faith* to it. (This idea of "faith" is very present in the work of Paul Goodman. My purpose here is not to address this issue; I only wish to say that belief is attached to the past, to lived experiences and the representations that are built based on these experiences, while faith is oriented toward what comes next, what is yet to come.)

My faith is that every word, every feeling, every gesture, every action is aimed at others. They are created by and for others. Active and passive, in the middle voice as Perls and Goodman would say. They are events *of* the field, not only *in* a field.

This is what we may call "intentionality". This concept was coined by Brentano, the grandfather of phenomenology, and picked up and refined by Husserl as a characteristic of consciousness. In order to extend this concept from the realm of philosophy to that of psychology, I had to stretch it somewhat, following Merleau-Ponty's example in doing so.

This intentionality is not only a purely mental fact, as could be the case in Husserl's work, but rather a wider experience: a bodily experience, and more specifically an expressive experience, which leads me to refer to it as "intentionality in flesh and blood".

Of course, intentionality is vague, confused and sometimes even chaotic before it is narrowed down into a real "intention", which is probably more explicit and conscious. But I am discussing intentionality, not intention. Intentionality is "upstream" while intention is "downstream".

This stage of gestalt formation is somewhat neglected. In fact, it is the very beginning of any process, the earliest phase of experience. The facts mentioned above (affects, emotions, actions, words, gestures, etc.), if they are approached from a purely individualistic perspective, will only be *premature differentiations*. Similarly, the gestalt therapist who asks the patient to take responsibility for what he feels can accentuate this premature differentiation by inducing a responsibility that is itself also premature.

In a two-person psychology – a field perspective – attention must be paid to the situation, and every feeling, sensation, action, expression, gesture, etc. must be regarded as belonging to the situation before being assigned to any differentiated individuals. Very quickly, of course, each participant appropriates everything he is used to considering himself according to his habits, patterns, character, memories and personality function. This is how the system of self-representations continues existing and unceasingly confirming itself.

This way of thinking is reinforced by our habit of understanding or explaining any situation based on what happened earlier in someone's personal history.

Let us remind ourselves of an ancient little Taoist tale, which illustrates yet another paradigm shift:

> This Chinese story is about a farmer who lived in a poor village in the country-side. People thought he was very lucky because he had a horse that he used for working in the fields and travelling. One day his horse ran away. All its neighbours lamented his misfortune, but the farmer simply said, "Maybe!"
>
> A few days later the horse returned, accompanied by two wild horses. The neighbours then rejoiced in his luck but the farmer simply said, "Maybe!"
>
> The next day the farmer's son tried to ride one of the wild horses, but the horse threw him to the ground and broke his leg. Neighbours expressed their sympathy to the farmer in light of this misfortune, but the farmer only said, "Maybe!"
>
> The following week, a group of recruitment officers came to the village to press-gang the young men into the army because of the war. They rejected the farmer's son because of his broken leg. When the neighbours told him how lucky he was, the farmer replied, "Maybe!"

Among the various possible meanings that can be drawn from this story, I would like to highlight one in particular: the meaning of an experience is built – or can be built – in relation to the future or the "next", not the past. Of course we could go on and on about the host of past circumstances that may have caused the horse to run away: the fence around its pasture that wasn't high enough or strong enough, the farmer who hadn't been watchful enough because of this or that, etc.

But this story shows how the future provides meaning, to the point where any desire to reference the past fades away out of lack of interest. Couldn't we see this as a potential direction for psychotherapeutic practice?

An epistemological tradition links the construction of meaning to history, in a more or less linear sense, and this mode is almost considered scientific. Although one may doubt its scientific nature, it can be regarded as the clinical attitude par excellence. Sometimes this clinical attitude proves quite close to the psychothera-peutic position. Nonetheless, I maintain that the clinical attitude and the psycho-therapeutic attitude are rooted in two starkly dissimilar approaches. For proof, one need only open a few books on the clinical, phenomenological approach to find detailed descriptions of patients, their behaviours and symptoms, their affects and their world, without ever questioning how this knowledge is constituted. The observer and the clinician are completely absent from the picture, and the patient is reified through the eyes of an expert who willingly denies the parameters of his encounter with him. There again, the method remains that of a single-person psy-chology, and it is reasonable to question its relevance in the realm of psychotherapy.

Even Freud, a year before his death, published a somewhat visionary article entitled "Constructions in Analysis" in which he no longer claimed to be so sure that the analyst's role is to *discover* a past covered by the strata of years. We may recall that his favourite metaphor compared the analyst's work with that of the archaeologist. It became quite clear to him that the search for the "truth" of mean-ing was perhaps not as important as the therapeutic relevance of meanings that could be "constructed". Paul Goodman himself, when discussing this issue, regu-larly uses the phrase "discovering-and-inventing", referring to the possible dual direction of therapeutic work.

Based on these considerations, let us return to the question of intentionality and try to see how we can approach it, knowing that despite its vague and cha-otic nature, it structures the field of experience. At this level, the therapist's aes-thetic function will most likely be called upon: his or her ability to contribute to the formation of forms that will be set in motion. Merleau-Ponty calls our atten-tion to "speaking words": speech that is in a nascent state (*in status nascendi*) and animated by a significant intention, which attempts to "put into words a silence that precedes it", to quote Merleau-Ponty (1964, p. 166). He distinguishes it from what he calls "spoken speech", which is based on layered meanings and "can draw on available meanings like on an acquired fortune" (1945, p. 229). Using these acquired, available meanings, the creator (in the same way as a child) knows how to produce other acts of expression, reconverting spoken speech into newly expres-sive speech. Interested readers may refer to Chapter 7 of *Gestalt Therapy*, in which Goodman discusses verbalizing and poetry.

Recounting Experience

In the non-dualistic perspective of gestalt therapy – that is to say, by positioning ourselves beyond what Perls and Goodman called "false dichotomies" such as that between body and mind – nothing can be thought outside of what the body feels. It would therefore be inconsistent to separate or oppose a deliberate or thought-out intentionality and bodily intentionality, even though the latter may exist outside the field of consciousness. Our approach focuses on what the patient says is present in his or her immediate awareness. Beyond this limit, psychotherapy helps broaden one's field of awareness to the realms of sensations, emotions, feelings, actions, behaviours, thoughts, memories, representations, fantasies, perceptions of the environment, etc.

The first phase of constructing the gestalt involves allowing a clear figure to emerge or develop, which can then be deployed. By "raking together" partial experiences that we are immediately aware of with other experiences that have just begun to emerge, we reassemble this experience and put it into conflict or dialogue in a single direction of meaning. Every practitioner knows to what extent exposing the coincidence between an anecdote related by the patient, the bodily experience associated with it, the accompanying gestures, etc. structures a substantially different orientation than that which could be triggered by words alone (intentionality which is verbalized and thus becomes intention) which are pronounced, sometimes without any regard to the situation.

If intentionality "directs itself towards", its meaning must be sought in the overall situation: in the field understood as a "structure of possibilities" (Deleuze, quoted by Miller, 2002); these possibilities cannot be reduced to the "organism" alone, or even to the psyche alone, to which too many clinicians attempt to limit it.

Intuition

Clinicians often use the term "intuition" to describe the modality that has allowed them to access the other and thereby enabled them to conduct an intervention, which is occasionally relevant. Although some would remind us that this modality of accessing the other is not exempt from attributions of meaning or projections, or even counter-transference issues, it nevertheless provides knowledge (which is often unrepresentable and ineffable) of certain elements of the patient's experience.

My hypothesis is that this intuition is formed in situ, at the crossroads of perception and resonance. The practitioner's self-knowledge, developed through his or her own personal therapy and supervision, allows him or her to clarify certain components of resonance that can play a role in the process. The rest of the task involves returning to what has been perceived, sometimes unconsciously, and very quickly summarized in a process that may seem passive. Which signals – linguistic, bodily, vocal, sub-vocal, contextual or atmospheric – are perceived by the clinician and immediately blended into a comprehensive, implicit meaning?

It is important to recall that intuitions – like perceptions – are also organized by the clinician's knowledge, expertise and experience. I would probably not have the intuition to sense that a certain person was full of shame from which he sought to defend himself, that he may have been the victim of abuse and mistreatment, or that his depression was the result of some skeleton in the closet or a ghost of his past, if the theories involved were totally foreign to my way of thinking.

Encountering Another Intentionality

The central postulation of gestalt therapy is based on contact. The human being is fundamentally contact: creative or conservative adjustment in an environment. Intentionality exists both in and through otherness. The therapeutic encounter is a meeting of intentionalities, each one encountering the other and thereby refining it. Through the encounter, intentionalities take on the form of intentions.

In a previous study (Robine, 2001), I called upon the concept of affordance to broaden the spectrum of linguistic options that would allow me to speak in terms of field and not only according to the solipsistic concept. This neologism was coined by Gibson (1979), the founder of eco-psychology, based on the verb "to afford": to have the means to do something. It designates a characteristic that refers to both "the organism" and "the environment": to the fundamental properties that determine how "the object" can be used. A chair provides support; its affordance allows me to consider sitting, in relation to my intentions, perceptions and possibilities.

Affordance is at work in a therapy session, as in any situation. The patient perceives the psychotherapist and his or her affordance, which activates certain ways in which the patient can "use" the therapist and deactivates others. My perception of a chair can trigger the desire to sit down; if I need to access an object out of reach at the top of my bookshelf, I will perceive a number of affordances in the situation, such as a chair or a box to stand on. I may even arrange unusual affordances: perceiving a pile of phonebooks as something to stand on or seeing someone in the room as perhaps being able to give me a leg up to reach the top shelf. Contact with my environment reveals me to myself and exposes some of my potentialities, at the same time as I endow my environment with potentialities that were perhaps hitherto unexplored. Nevertheless, these functions take into account the object's possible affordance: I will not perceive the calculator on my desk as a possible means of accessing the shelf out of reach. "Situations do not cause our actions, but they do not represent a simple background against which we realize our intentions, either. We only perceive a situation according to our aptitudes and our current preparedness to act", wrote Joas (1992). In the therapeutic encounter, each of us is the essential constituent element of the situation for the other, both consciously and unconsciously.

The Other Affects Me

Both common sense and shared experience allow me to recognize that the other affects me when I am in his presence. He affects me, which means that he makes me feel, imagine, think, infer, experience physically and emotionally, etc. Even my neutrality (if such a thing exists) or my indifference are not the pure products of my will or my choices. My experience is a connection. It is connected to my intentionality, of course, but also to the presence of the other and to his own target.

My working hypothesis is that awareness of what I experience in the here and now of the situation is an effective tool for gaining knowledge of the other's intentionality. I am tempted to connect this assertion to what Perls and Goodman said about emotion:

> An emotion is the integrative awareness of a relation between the organism and the environment. As such, it is a function of the field. [. . .] In the sequence of grounds and figures, the emotions take over the motivational force of the urges and appetites [. . .] [They] are means of cognition. [. . .] [T]hey are unique deliveries of the state of the organism/environment field . . .
>
> (Perls, Hefferline & Goodman, 1951, 407–408)

My feeling in the other's presence is thus an indicator of what is in the field: it says something about me, about the other, about the situation, about the atmosphere, about our encounter. I fully agree with Perls and Goodman when they recognize that as a type of cognition, emotions are fallible, but that we can correct, cultivate and refine them (and especially, I would add, we can talk about them as clues to what is there).

When a woman I accompany in group therapy begins speaking confusedly, almost incoherently, accompanied by various vegetative manifestations, onomatopoeia and babbling, the more I try to understand her, the less I understand her. The only information I can cling to at that particular moment is my experience that gradually takes the form of a desire to hold her in my arms as I could do with a child, and at the same time the desire to beat her! When I manage to put a name to what happened to her, she calms down and begins to talk about the abuse she suffered as a child, which she had never mentioned before: an experience of violence and tenderness intertwined. Her intentionality, or that of the situation, was pushing her confusedly in this direction of meaning.

Conscious and Unconscious Intentionality

For those who work with gestalt therapy, I don't think it makes sense to rely on a distinction between what other approaches may classify as conscious or unconscious at the level of intentionality, another dissociation which is now ranked among the "false dichotomies" described by Perls and Goodman. Our approach, which focuses on becoming aware, does not require the premise of a "place" where potentially contradictory intentions may arise and confront those of which one is already aware. As such, the symptom must not be overlooked when dealing with the issue of an intentional purpose, which must bring conscious and unconscious experience together and unfold them in order to explain it. A child who suddenly starts to fail his classes at school is certainly not aware that by doing so he is aiming to direct his mother's attention and supportive presence toward him, thereby preventing her from slipping further into a state of depression. However, as long as intentionality is not exposed – which does not necessarily involve becoming aware of it – and as long as other methods of achieving this key objective are not developed, the symptom will persist, waiting to be recognized.

For this reason, when we start to work on unfolding the symptom, I consider it fundamental to expose its impact on the environment: how it may be felt, how it affects others, and how it triggers reactions. This information is essential in order to venture any guesses about the meaning of one's intentionality.

Gestalt therapy states that when a symptom is formed, it starts out as a creative adjustment to the situation – an attempt to solve the problem, albeit a clumsy one – thereby implicitly recognizing the intentionality of this symptom. It is an intended meaning that has been addressed.

I would therefore situate intentionality as a constituent of the emergence of the figure and consequently related to the "id of the situation" – to its ". . . and then" – in a field perspective. If, as I suggest, individuation is to be found by exposing the reflections of this intentionality, in a clinical situation I can only approach it through interactions with the patient, which may be vague or confusing. Only by moving upstream from deliberate intentions towards this imprecise intentionality – which says as much about itself as it does about the other and the situation – can we free the self from part of the game of representations predetermined by the personality function, providing access to an ego mode that is firmly linked to the id of the situation.

From this initial chaos, which may be vague or confusing, this present or regained confluence and this predifferentiation found upstream from premature differentiations, the dynamics of individuation are based on forming, identifying and recognizing intention. If we accept a field hypothesis – and thus one of situated activity and situated speech – then vague intentionality (which starts out as nothing more than direction of meaning) will offer much more to discover and/or invent concerning speaking speech than spoken speech; at the very least we will seek speaking speech in spoken speech.

The body "is not only an expressive space among all the others, but the very origin of all the others – the very movement of expression, [. . .] a primordial operation of meaning where what is expressed does not exist independently of the expression" (Merleau-Ponty, 1945, pp. 171 & 193). Meaning drives my body just as it drives my developing speech. Intentionality and corporeality awaken each other. It is not through clear meanings or developed thought that others communicate with me or that I communicate with them at first, but rather a certain bodily way of being: speaking speech, whether verbal or nonverbal. And my welcoming of the intentionality of others is not consciously thought-over or explicit, but rather a certain mode of my existence in the mode of "the affected being".

"The communication or comprehension of gestures is obtained through the reciprocity of my intentions and the other's actions, of my gestures and the intentions readable in the other's conduct. Everything occurs as if the other's intention inhabited my body or as if my intentions inhabited his. The gesture that I witness sketches an intentional object. This object becomes present and is fully understood when my body's powers adjust to it and cover it. The gesture lies before me as a question; it shows me certain sensitive parts of the world and invites me to join it there," wrote Merleau-Ponty beautifully (1945, pp. 215–216).

It is not so much the words or representations that establish the first communication, but rather a significant intention that triggers speech and bodily movement in an implicit register. Someone is with the patient and, in an act that may be either conscious or unconscious, an intentionality targets and affects him. This is why the groping attempt to verbalize how the other affects me reflects a number of clues that can help expose its implicit target and thereby help differentiate it.

The body's expressiveness should be distinguished from the intention of meaning. Meaning consists in using a sign to designate an object and communicate its meaning to an other. Expressing does not involve the intermediary of a sign. Smiling is not a sign that refers to a meaning: it is the bodily mode of meaning, the intentionality experienced by the subject which becomes meaning when it is perceived and responded to by others.

The bodily experience of a subject is rarely independent of the intentionality that it entails. I invite the reader to test this statement by carrying out a very simple little experiment: start by holding your hands in front of you, carefully focusing your attention on your fingers, and very gently touch the tip of your left index finger with your right index finger. Keep in mind the distinct sensations that you feel in each of your index fingers. Next, perform the gesture in the opposite order: touch the tip of your right index finger with your left index finger. You will no doubt notice that at the moment of contact, each index finger feels differently depending on whether it is driven by the intentionality of "touching" or "being touched". From a purely mechanical point of view, the feeling should be the same, but when the touched finger becomes the touching finger, the difference is clearly structured by a specificity of intentionality rather than any objectified factors.

Nevertheless, the only access I can have to the intentionality of others is linked to their expressiveness. "In each system, the other can be defined a priori by his or her expressive (i.e. implicit, enveloping) value. [. . .] The other cannot be separated from the expressiveness that constitutes him or her. [. . .] To understand the other as such, we were entitled to claim special conditions of experience [. . .] the moment when what is expressed does not yet exist (to us) beyond what it expresses", insists Deleuze (1968a, pp. 334–335), even adding, "We must understand that the other is not a structure among others in the field of perception. He or she is the structure that affects the entire field and the way the whole thing functions" (Deleuze, 1969a, p. 58).

Phenomenology has taught us that it is impossible to separate things from the way they appear to someone. This hypothesis is radically different from the belief that the therapist is neutral, and invites us to instead consider the ways in which each of these things appear to him or her as components of the phenomenon itself. Far from lamenting my subjectivity, including the role it may have in determining the organization of the field, I claim my "being affected" as a tool for understanding others. Braque said that the painter did not seek to "reconstitute an anecdotal fact but rather to constitute a pictorial fact" (1948, p. 30). By analogy, I would say that the therapist does not attempt to reconstitute an anecdotal fact but rather to constitute a therapeutic fact.

We have thus moved away from a purportedly scientific approach to fully embrace an aesthetic approach. If I want to understand (note that I say understand, not explain) and feel the light, should I turn to physicists, who talk about photons and wave phenomena, or to the paintings of artists from centuries past? The therapeutic situation is a situation of taking shape, construction and deconstruction of forms (gestalts) in and by the encounter between two intentionalities, which may be conflicting.

Provisional Conclusion

Many philosophical, sociological, psychological or psychotherapeutic approaches have placed the notion of the subject at the core of their theories and practices. Our thought patterns are built on this assumption. In these approaches, the self (or subject, etc. – whatever one wishes to call it) is under house arrest because it has been confused with the individual. It is therefore locked up and alienated. In the 1940s and 50s, the emerging gestalt therapy launched a theory for psychotherapy that rushed into the cracks that this system of thought had begun to show. The cracks became breaches, which became faults, and then a paradigm shift took place. Everything was to be rebuilt in a field perspective: therapy was rethought as situation, practice as an encounter and expression as an effect of the field before being a manifestation of a psyche of which it is more a generator than a consequence.

In the therapeutic encounter, both might be tempted to position themselves as a priori established or individuated. This method has been proven over the course of decades. Another method may arise from the foundations laid by our founders and their definition of self. The self, a catalyst of the functions required to make contact with novelty and make creative adjustments, is engaged in the situation. The gestalt therapist is engaged in the situation and this engagement is part of the field's very structure. He or she affects others and is affected by others. The implicit intention of each participant may be babbled, based on each individual's experience in his or her feelings and perceptions. In this respect, the moment of pre-contacting, emergence and/or construction of the figure is critical. It makes it possible to navigate what is the same, known or part of the narrative, but also to depart from an undifferentiated whole which will have to undergo continuous, unending individuation. The therapist is one of the facts of the situation and his or her intentionality will simply be to open up conditions of possibility. Forms of this possibility will have to be created.

Context: This article was written for Actua Psy, *the journal published by the SNPPsy in 2004. The Syndicat National des Praticiens en Psychothérapie et Psychanalyse was one of the first, if not the first, professional organization created in France in 1981 to organize, promote and defend the profession of psychotherapist. I have been involved since its foundation and wrote this article when the SNPPsy asked me to introduce the evolution of gestalt therapy, which until then had been known to the wider public and to professionals of other approaches, especially in its intrapsychic form promoted by F. Perls in California in the late 1960s.*

Chapter 2

Self, Artist of Contact

I

More than sixty-five years ago, Perls and Goodman introduced a turning point in psychotherapy with *Gestalt Therapy* (hereafter designated PHG [Perls, Hefferline and Goodman], 1951). With many of their proposals – which have most likely still not yet been sufficiently developed – they anticipated many later developments in the social sciences. This is particularly true for the concept of self, which was displaced, decentred and then relocated and temporalized. At the time, so-called modern psychology – a solipsistic discipline if ever there was one – recognized only an individualized self as the sole "reality", and the psyche was one of its main variations. Based on "the simplest and first reality" – namely that no human function exists without contact with the environment – the authors structured a fundamentally innovative way of thinking and praxis, in direct contact with this natural conception of human nature. This fundamental human activity – which consists in establishing and modulating contact with one's environment; bringing out and constructing adapted, creative figures from the novelty of each situation; deconstructing any completed or obsolete figures – is the limited but essential function they assign to the self.

If the founders attribute to the self the task of activating and synthesizing the functions it is necessary to engage in a creative contact with the environment, it is clear that the self exists only *when* and *where* there is contact: an ephemeral function, a function of varying intensity depending on the difficulty presented by the field. Under this conception, there is no claim that the self existed beforehand and reveals, manifests or expresses itself in contact; instead, it *is* contact; it is created in and through contact. In a field defined as "an organism and its environment", the self-function designates the internal movements of this field: movements of integration and differentiation, unification and individuation, action and transformation . . . To grow and develop, the organism must encounter what is new, different, not itself; it makes it into a figure – that is to say, it forms a Gestalt – and in the operation of contact that it thereby carries out, driven by the excitement accompanying this formation of forms, it returns to this continued individuation, this unceasing self/world differentiation. This process is called self. "[Self] is only a small factor

DOI: 10.4324/9781003515760-3

in the total organism/environment interaction, but it plays the crucial role of finding and making the meanings that we grow by" (PHG, 1951, Chapter 1, §11).

This relocation of the self and its repositioning as a field phenomenon may seem astonishing due to its prophetic nature, pre-empting the work of many philosophers, sociologists and essayists of the second half of the 20th century. However, the attentive reader of *Gestalt Therapy* will notice certain oscillations between a traditional conception of a self-entity – sometimes called a "self-object" by some later authors – and the innovative design they sketched out, and with it a new paradigm that would be developed in diverse forms – often less radical than the original – by several authors of postmodernity, social constructionism, intersubjective psychoanalysis or other identity theorists.

II

In my native language (French), the concept of self cannot be translated by any exact equivalent. Some authors choose to translate "self" as "*soi*", thereby reducing it to a more conventional concept. In *Gestalt Therapy*, while "self" refers to the function of the field mentioned above, in the same text it is also used to designate the sedimentation that may take place in the aftermath of creative organism/environment contacts and in this case, "*soi*" may be an appropriate translation. English seems to be one of the rare languages in which "self" can refer to both the process and its result.

Several authors – in particular the British philosopher Stephen E. Toulmin (1977) – have shown that in the English language "self" originally existed only as a suffix (e.g. "myself") or a prefix (e.g. "self-control"), emphasizing its fundamentally reflexive nature, until the relatively recent point when the word found itself isolated, nominalized and therefore theorized as a noun. William James (1890) and later George H. Mead (1934) probably played the biggest role in turning this prefix/suffix into a separate concept. In most other languages, this reflexive process and its result cannot be designated by a single concept. As a result, it can be difficult for gestalt therapists from other cultures to appropriate the use of this concept.

In my language, this reflexive character is expressed by two pronouns: "*je*" ("I"), which designates the verbal agent, and "*me*" or "*moi*" ("me" or "myself"), which designates the beneficiary or receiver of the action carried out by "*je*". We call this form the "reflexive voice", as in "*je me promène*" ("I walk" but literally "I walk myself") or "*je me lave les dents*" ("I brush my teeth" but literally "I wash myself the teeth"). (This is the same reflexive form that will be used to express retroflection.) One of the three essential properties that Perls, Hefferline and Goodman attribute to the self is the *middle voice* (which they mistakenly call "the middle mode" since in grammar, "mode" refers to the indicative, the subjunctive, the participle, etc.) in reference to ancient Greek grammar, which has this form of conjugating verbs (and thus actions) without the need for differentiated pronouns (PHG, 1951, Chapter 10, §4). The two other properties they focus on are *spontaneity* and *engagement in the situation*, which we will return to later on.

III

How can we use a concept that has barely any roots in a given culture? If self, with its two meanings – process and structure – does not correspond to an equivalent definition in another language, how can this term find its place in the clinician's vernacular "toolbox", to borrow an expression from Foucault (1972)?

In fact, in daily practice, drafting session notes, during supervision and in the thoughts of the practitioner in action, the concept of self is hardly present. But Perls and Goodman provided a description of its functions and its dynamics which makes up a set of valuable, operative beacons. In the same way that physicists can describe light sometimes as particles and sometimes as waves, the clinician can address the self sometimes by turning its partial structures (also called functions) into figures and sometimes by tracking its temporal deployment (also called contact sequence or construction/deconstruction of a Gestalt).

Self is thus a unifying concept that brings together the ingredients required to enable the creative adjustment of an organism and its environment. "For the most part the self creates special structures for special purposes [. . .] The subject-matter of a formal psychology would be the exhaustive classification, description and analysis of the possible structures of the self. (This is the subject-matter of Phenomenology)" (PHG, 1951, Chapter 10, §5).

As such, I believe – and am aware that this is a choice on my part – that the theory proposed by our founding book need not be approached as a metapsychology but rather as a *theory of practice*, or even *a theory* for *a specific practice*, based on an anthropology, a conception of man in the world. As in philosophy, it is possible to differentiate between *metaphysical* approaches and *phenomenological* approaches, and the psychological movement that Perls and Goodman belonged to proposes to develop based on what is observed at the organism/environment contact boundary, not metapsychological inferences or speculative preconceptions.

I have often had occasion to denounce the pan-explanatory hegemonic temptation to apply certain theoretical systems to a field that is not theirs (Robine, 2004, 2011a). On the contrary, I am in favour of placing different frames of reference in dialectical tension with one another, without looking for a truth that, in any event, will always escape us.

IV

Our cultural tendency urges us to reify the self, place it at the heart of the individual, define its outline and provide it with attributes – some of which are supposedly "true" and others "false". Yet, as we mentioned, "It is a reflexive operation by which the actor is specified, limited and defined. This operation presupposes integration into a field to achieve ongoing differentiation. It is individuation, not the individual. It is Montaigne's 'I do not paint the being; I paint the passage' (1580/1969)" (Robine, 2004/2012). The self is unfolding, in flux, constantly evolving, becoming by connecting, through its contacts with its human and non-human environment.

Our authors study three partial structures of the self (which, they regretted, were often taken for the overall functioning of the self) which "are the major stages of creative adjustment" (PHG, 1951, Chapter 19, §5).

It should be noted that for Perls and Goodman, there can be no question of reducing the self to these three functions alone: they choose to limit their focus to these three because they are essential to organizing the figure/background process; in other words, they are the three functions that act in implementing an adapted, creative contact.

These three partial structures of the self (or functions) are called personality-function, id-function and ego-function, names that condense the ideas they refer to: the self functioning in ego mode, the self functioning in personality mode, etc.

The id-function means "the given background dissolving into its possibilities, including organic excitations and past unfinished situations becoming aware, and the environment vaguely perceived, and the inchoate feelings connecting organism and environment" (ibid.).

The personality-function "is the created figure that the self becomes and assimilates to the organism, uniting it with the results of previous growth" (ibid.).

The ego-function is "the progressive identification with and alienation of the possibilities, the limiting and heightening of the ongoing contact, including motor behaviour, aggressing, orientation and manipulation" (ibid.).

V

Although gestalt therapy theorists always take the precaution of attaching the term "function" to each of these partial structures so that their definitions are not confused with those used in psychoanalysis, many regret that they still contain psychoanalytical terms – "id" and "ego" in particular.

"Id" refers to the function of the self that manifests needs, desires, appetites, impulses . . . It is the direction of meaning. Given that this moment of the experience is lived in a subverbal mode, the body is its expression – or, to alter Freud's well-known formulation, one could say that the body is the "royal road" to access the id. But the road should not be confused with what it leads to . . . It is more *awareness* than *consciousness* that grants us access to the ephemeral contents of the id-function, if indeed it can be addressed independently of other functions.

Although the terms are not fully superimposable – far from it, in fact – I am tempted to address this moment of the experience using the term *intentionality*. Returning to Husserl:

Intentionality is an essential peculiarity of the sphere of mental processes taken universally in so far as all mental processes in some manner or other share in it; nevertheless, we cannot say of *each* mental process that it has intentionality [. . .] Intentionality is what characterizes *consciousness* in the pregnant sense and which, at the same time, justifies designating the whole stream of mental processes as the stream of consciousness and as the unity of *one* consciousness.

(Husserl, 1913/1950, p. 283)

Transferring such an important, widely commented concept from the philosophical sphere to the psychological sphere is, admittedly, risky business (Robine, 2004). I attribute the characteristic of the *implicit* to intentionality, and will reserve the *explicit* for [deliberate] intention. I thereby establish the same difference and the same relationship between intentionality and intention as the one that may exist between creativity and creation. Creativity – potential and direction of meaning – can only be exercised or perceived through a creation, which is a reduction of the possible forms in which creativity could manifest itself.

History has taught us that the dissemination of the concept of "ego" in the psychological sciences seems attributable to the English translator of Freud, who saw fit to translate Freud's "*Ich*" as "*Ego*", and this Ego was adopted by the francophone tradition, which translated it as "*Moi*". And that is how, if we think back to the distinction mentioned earlier between the "I" and the "me", the "me" would become the agent, instead of being the beneficiary or result of the action! It would therefore be wise, given the very definition of the "ego-function" provided by our founders and when it occurs in the experience, to restore its name to "*I*" or "*I-function*". It is indeed the function of the self, which is also ephemeral, which is responsible for selection and rejection, and the construction of the figure, i.e. the ongoing contact.

And the attribution of the *Ego* could fall on the personality-function, since this "I" is made up of sedimentations of successive experiences. But I do not deny the tradition that uses "personality" to refer to the set of characteristics of a particular individual, although PHG emphasize the difference between "who I am" and "who I think I am". And it is more this second aspect that defines the personality-function.

In his unpublished teachings, Isadore From stated that the ego-function was the bridge between the personality-functions or between the id and the environment; in other words, this ego-function could not get involved without support from one of the other two functions.

VI

A simplistic reading of these functions could lead some gestalt therapists to try to make their patients' words fit within the narrow framework of these partial structures as one might do with independent entities. Thus, if the patient described herself or stated one of her characteristics ("I am someone who . . ."), the therapist would diagnose a manifestation of the personality-function; a patient who stated his desire or need – or even ahead of that possibility, who expressed a bodily feeling – would be interpreted as driven by the id-function; a patient who made a choice would be seen as manifesting the exercise of her ego-function. This conception of a subject as made up of "little boxes" that are more or less sealed is far from meeting with my approval, since all experience mobilizes the entire self, and the therapist's focus on one partial function or another is related to the work that takes place from one moment to the next.

An expression that might "traditionally" be read as an expression of the personality-function could thus be used in work to build up access to the id-function, if such an orientation seems relevant. An amusing example can be imagined based on something Perls often said at his Esalen seminars: "I believe that I am the best therapist for any type of neurosis in the States, maybe in the world" (1969a; 1969b). If this statement were taken at face value, it might reveal the traits of a personality that is, at the very least, not character-ized by modesty. But the choice of organization of how the message is heard by the recipient can lead that listener down other paths: "What is this Perls trying to accomplish by having me hear this representation he has of himself? What does he want from me?" And in this way a focus placed on the id-function of the self can come to the foreground.

The concepts put forth to approach the deployment of the self can thus be used more dynamically and less structurally to serve as a gateway to the experience lived from moment to moment.

In addition, although the various functions of the self described by our authors can be addressed as partial structures, they can also be regarded as specific moments of the experience, as momentary dominant features in the course of building a Gestalt.

VII

The second way of looking at the self involves its temporal dimension. This modal-ity is described by the founders as a *sequence*: a succession or sequence of opera-tions that may lead to a phenomenological observation. In its so-called subsequent developments, this sequence was renamed "cycle" by certain schools of thought, which to me seems to be a completely inappropriate term. A cycle describes a recurring – and thus predictable – phenomenon such as the cycle of the seasons, the menstrual cycle, the cycle of the tides and the lunar cycle. This is – let us hope – far from being the case of the human experience and the creation of figure/background relations which lead to novelty and therefore the unknown.

This sequence is also described in terms of "process". In this regard, it seems important to consider the difference between "process" and "sequence". A process is defined by two basic characteristics: first of all, it is an ordered sequence that leads to a result. We can thus describe the series of operations that allows us, for example, to cook an egg or to complete an apprenticeship; the objective is specific and clearly defined. The second characteristic of a process is that the phenomena that follow one another in time present a coherent unity with the objective. Boiling water is part of the egg-cooking process, as is immersing the eggs in the water. But if during this operation I answer the phone or set the table, these actions are not part of the egg-cooking process, yet they are actually part of the sequence – that is to say, the series of my actions. Thus, during a therapy session – one of whose lines of work may concern "interruptions of contact" – is it more operative to focus on the process or on the sequence? In fact, we can only really know a process once it has been completed, since it then becomes possible to show the series of operations that contributed to its completion, without retaining parasitic or irrelevant parallel actions. However, these so-called parasitic actions that occur during contact and the construction of a Gestalt will not be absent from subsequent dysfunctions or even their attachment in a psychopathological form.

During a group therapy session, Pierre discusses his difficulty in accessing bodily sensations and the fact that, on the rare occasions when they do reach his consciousness, he cannot make sense of them and does not know what to do with them.

Work begins, focused on the consciousness of his bodily experience and, supported by the safety of the group setting and his trust in our contact, he manages to emerge and name sensations, not without some anxiety. Explicitly, the next moment appears to be a search for meaning and direction in contacting rooted in these sensations.

He pauses, then reports that something is happening in his mouth and that before continuing he would like to eat a piece of candy. He looks for the basket where the group organizer had set out a selection of sweets.

I draw his attention to this "need" to swallow something, just when the possibility of an action of expression was opening up – that is to say, the opposite movement, directed toward the world, not turned back toward the organism.

He asks for my support to experience this other possibility, suddenly aware of his propensity to interrupt at this specific point in the process by "swallowing" his feelings.

I suggest that he use his breathing – especially exhaling – to experience how it feels when he turns "something" rooted in his bodily sensations toward the world. Then, while remaining at a distance, I invite him to direct his breath in my direction, as if he wanted to hit me in the face with his exhalation. After a few breaths, emotion accompanies his breathing; the feeling of being welcomed opens access to the other, to the world, and the sequence can continue in the novelty of this mode of contact.

This illustration shows how a mini-event – which appears to be a parasite to the process – takes its place in the sequence. It also reveals how the "status" that the therapist assigns to the event can be decisive. The current concept of "interrupting the contact" – which should obviously be understood to mean "interrupting the figure of contact being constructed" and not "interrupting the contact between you and me" – therefore strikes me as highly ambiguous. I am more inclined to entertain the hypothesis that contact (the construction of the figure) continues despite appearances by taking on a form whose "logic" may escape me but which should be considered connected to the experience. The interruption may thus be caused by the therapist following the *process* rather than the *sequence*.

VIII

This sequence has been described multiple times throughout the history of gestalt therapy. In my view, the description provided by Perls and Goodman is still fully relevant insofar as it addresses the sequence in terms of figure/background relationships rather than in behavioural terms as was generally the case later on. They highlight how each phase is characterized by a specific figure, supported by a background that is no less specific, and thus creates a kind of dance between figures that advance into the foreground and then return to the background, enriching it and enabling the establishment of a brighter, clearer, sharper figure. What is offered is thus a true aesthetics of the self: a description of the formation of forms (*Gestaltung*).

It does not seem necessary, within the framework and limits of this chapter, to detail how the sequence of the deployment of the self unfolds, since this is extensively discussed in Chapters XII and XIII of PHG (PHG, 1951). Let us only briefly review its theoretical choreography:

Initially there is creative undifferentiation, that moment where nothing constitutes a figure and where the permanence of the background is ensured by the body. (Here I am of course speaking of the "phenomenal body" as theorized by Merleau-Ponty in his first book (1945) and which he later came to call "flesh" (1964).) Then the situation opens up to the emergence of sensations outside of this undifferentiated background. The figure, driven by the background, is then constituted by the direction of meaning (desire, need, appetite, urge, etc.). This is the forecontact phase. The figure joins the background, melting into it. The background is no longer just "body" but becomes what might be called a "desiring body", and the "possible objects" to contact are built into figures (others, objects, contacts, meanings, experiences, environment, etc.). The "I" is at work making choices and rejections. The choices – and then THE choice – refine the figure. Rejected hypotheses move into the background, thereby feeding it. This is the contacting phase. Next, what made up the direction of meaning can blend momentarily into the chosen "object". This is the final contact phase, a term which recalls that this contact, this construction of a figure was aimed at reaching this *final purpose*. But it is not the *end* of the sequence, since the time has now come for withdrawal and the assimilation of the experience. What has been experienced with "the chosen object" joins the background and the experience enriches the self's personality-function. The figure gradually fades away until it disappears as such. This is the post-contact phase.

This sequence, which I have oversimplified here, can be criticized due to its relatively solipsistic description. It gives rise to various subsequent contributions to fit into the field paradigm, which places it in a perspective of co-creation. We will return to it when we discuss this paradigm.

IX

Approached in its temporal dimension, the self appears to be an ever-changing function: operating at very low intensity when the organism is at rest and only slightly mobilized when the situation is contacted through routines and systems of habit, the more difficult the field and the more it requires both adaptation and creativity, the more the self is fully engaged.

It is often described using the metaphor of the sea or the river ("We never bathe twice in the same river", wrote Heraclitus in the sixth century bce). Although it is mobilized in various ways and constantly created by the novelty of situations, the self is not multiple (in the sense of having multiple selves). The sea can be calm, choppy, stormy, warm or cold, with or without waves, turquoise or grey, but it will always be "the sea" because the word "sea" designates what unites all of these changing characteristics, whatever they may be. I see "the self" as the unifying principle of the forms of experience.

X

I would like to briefly mention what our founders called "interruptions of contact", which they only discussed in the last chapters of the founding book (PHG, 1951, Chapters 14 & 15). It should, however, be noted that these interruptions were the focus of most of the practical section written by Hefferline and Perls (PHG, 1951).

These modalities – confluence, introjection, projection, retroflection, egotism, repression, sublimation and reaction formation – have been the subject of much controversy in the community, concerning their names as much as their status in the theoretical apparatus. The *Gestalt Journal* amply documented this debate over the course of the 1990s. Incidentally, it should be noted that repression, sublimation and reaction formation seem to have fallen out of fashion – or been rejected? – by the majority of Gestalt clinicians, without having been the subject of a critical study.

Some currents of gestalt therapy place these modalities at the centre of therapeutic work, which may lead the therapist to engage in a real hunt for what they see as major disruptions. Moreover, for a long time, in a process initiated by Perls and amplified and expanded by the Polsters (Polster, E. & M. 1973/1983), these modalities were considered "resistances" before the theoretical error was recognized.

The term "interrupting the contact" manifests a certain ambiguity related to the implicit definition that each of us may have of contact. A human being is always in contact with something or someone, be it with the air he breathes or the ground on which he stands. Contact can move – even very rapidly – from one figure to another (in a sort of noematic change, to twist Husserl's term) just as it can change modalities, switching from visual contact to emotional contact, for example (which would be a noetic variation). This means that it is not "the contact" that is interrupted, but rather the object of the contact or the modality that is replaced by another. As I mentioned following the illustration quoted above, I can also hypothesize that the self engaged in a situation remains involved in a theme for longer than it may seem . . .

Since these modalities are described in two chapters entitled "Loss of ego-functions", Isadore From (1981ff.) gave them this name in the plural. His reading of this chapter led him to understand that when a subject presented disturbances of the id-function or the personality-function, the ego-function was no longer able to make healthy identifications and alienations, and was therefore momentarily lost. Then, in this absence of functioning in ego-mode, along came one of these modalities as a substitute (projection, introjection, etc.), an expression of dysfunction and therefore of pathology.

Another reading can also be made of the rhetoric of this chapter. What happens when there is a loss of the ego-function? When this is the case, what happens to the modalities of contact called introjection, projection, etc.? How do they operate *differently*? It is therefore no longer they themselves that are dysfunctional, but instead the experience in the absence of the self's ego-mode. Each of us could cite many examples of situations in which it felt "healthy" to retroflect or introject!

Another difficulty associated with these concepts is related to the confusion that can occur between these modalities – specific moments of the ongoing contact – and making them chronic. Introjection or retroflection designate operating modes during the course of a contact sequence, so *introject* or *retroflect*, for example, designate their fixation. This confusion, which is unfortunately quite common, leads some to speak of an *introjection* which, for example, is supposedly rooted in childhood experiences, whereas they are perhaps in the presence of "old" *introject* – the fixation of content and making it chronic – and certainly not an *introjecting* person. Psychopathology should be thought of in terms of calling on fixed forms rather than implementing a creative adjustment.

To give a categorical name to these modalities, in 1997 I proposed the term *"flexions"* found in the French translation of Binswanger's *Dream and Existence* (1930). This term, borrowed from linguistics, describes the way words (verbs or nouns) are conjugated or declined. It therefore has no pejorative or dysfunctional connotation: it only refers to derivations, variations related to the context. It seems to me that this concept lets us address these contact boundary phenomena as *variations* rather than symptoms. It helps us avoid focusing on these phenomena, unfolding instead them as gateways to the experience.

XI

In the preceding pages – aside from certain reservations, critiques or personal formulations – I tried to stay as close as possible to the original proposals of our founders. The occasionally solipsistic or intrapsychic dimension of certain statements will probably not have escaped the eye of an attentive reader.

In recent decades, a turning point occurred among a number of theorists and practitioners faced with the observation that although the field perspective was still always mentioned among the founding principles of gestalt therapy, for a long time gestalt therapy was far from being integrated into psychotherapeutic practice, which often remained individualistic. The field principle appeared to be more of a slogan than a reality, and our concepts needed to be revisited to allow a greater coherence to emerge.

When we launch this type of paradigm shift, it may therefore be appropriate to look at whether the conception of the self requires a few inflections, or even a redefinition.

The field that Perls and Goodman discuss is not a "thing": they call it the "organism/environment field". That means that every field is a field "of". There is always an organizing principle of the field: the eye's field of vision; a conscious being's field of consciousness; the field of psychology, with psychology taken to be the organizer of a field of knowledge; etc. (Robine, 2008).

Frank Staemmler (2006a) made a major contribution to clarifying this concept as discussed throughout the various sources and by all the different contributors, and also highlighted the inconsistencies and contradictions of successive authors' implicit or explicit definitions. Some would approach a conception of the field as an entity or a semi-entity, others as an experience – in the phenomenological sense – which is both continuous and transient. As with any attempt at theorization, there are choices to be made. For my part, I consider the field as an experience of interrelatedness between an organism and its environment, and prefer to try to use other concepts to designate other specific regards: context, situation, realm, milieu, background, environment, system, etc. What is certain is that none of us is immune to shifts in the use of the concept!

> When referring to contact and other field phenomena, Perls and Goodman periodically introduced the distinction between "in the field" and "of the field". Placing the subject, the body, the contact, etc. as events of the field and not in the field clarifies the matter by opposing the two major uses of the concept of field: one that results in reification and the other that maintains the field in flux.
>
> (Robine, 2004)

According to this conception, "field" is a paradigm that fundamentally defines a posture, a focus on how each of us can be created by our environment at the same time as we are creators of our environment. In one of his writings – I do not know which – Peter Philippson evoked the famous Escher drawing *Drawing Hands* which shows a hand drawing a hand, which itself is drawing the hand that is drawing it . . . A great metaphor!

In the context of psychotherapy, this means taking into account the process-related fact that the therapist is co-created by the encounter with her patient, just as the patient is co-created by the encounter with his therapist. What is felt by each person involved, the experience that unfolds, spoken words, sensory and motor patterns, memories summoned, fantasies, historical parallels, the constructions of meaning . . . are first of all products *of the situation*.

The starting point of my question on "the situation" is found in a small expression by Perls and Goodman when they are discussing "the id of the situation" (Robine, 2002). This is again not a contextualized id, the id *in* a situation that they are talking about, but "the id *of* the situation". Far from the theory of "internal" drives and forces that animate us, the source of the id is localized in the situation – a joint creation – to then give rise to a specific, differentiated, individuating feeling in each of the actors involved.

I use the term **situation** to designate the overall perception/proprioception of elements of the field of all the actors involved: a perception that allows them to structure the context of their encounter, give it meaning and implicitly define the modalities of their interaction. It is a space that is constructed and delimited by each of the actors, who are themselves simultaneously constructed by that space and by the definition they give it.

It is also important not to lose sight of the fact that acting and reacting to the situation means simultaneously acting with one's own memory and one's own emotions, since they are part of each participant's [organism/environment] field.

To articulate the concept of field with that of situation, I would say – perhaps only provisionally! – that the situation is created by the intersection of and interaction between the fields of each of the actors involved. Each participant's immediate and selective perception of the implicit organization of the field of all the actors involved organizes the situation. From the field of the actors involved emerge affordances (Gibson, 1979) and valences (Lewin, 1936, 1951) which combine to form the situation (see Chapter 17).

The idea of a "common field" seems to have spread in recent years, both among gestalt therapists (e.g. Francesetti, 2015) and certain psychoanalysts, following Baranger's founding article (1961), built upon in particular by Ferro et al. (2009). To designate what is referred to by the term "common field" – or one of its variants ("bi-personal field", "dynamic field", etc.) – I prefer to use that of the situation to avoid using the same concept to refer to two different approaches, since this "common" field cannot match the descriptions of the organism/environment field as proposed by Perls and Goodman. The idea of "common" could too easily be understood as "shared", or even "similar".

What is important, to quote Merleau-Ponty, is implementing the following conception:

> In the experience of dialogue, a common ground is constituted between me and another; my thought and his form a single fabric, my words and those of my interlocutor are called forth by the state of discussion and are inserted into a shared operation of which neither of us is the creator. Here there is a being-shared-by-two, and the other person is no longer for me a simple behavior in my transcendental field, nor for that matter am I a simple behavior in his. We are, for each other, collaborators in a perfect reciprocity: our perspectives slip into each other, we coexist through a single world.
>
> (1945, trans. Routledge 2012, p. 370)

From this perspective, the constantly renewed novelty of the situation is what organizes the experience, and therapeutic work focuses less on what *was* than on what *will happen*. The therapeutic situation is no longer a simple repetition of history, but instead a potential space-time opening up to transformation. Traditional causalist assumptions are reversed: it is neither the patient's past nor even the therapist's that gives form to the now, but instead the situation co-created in the now that may possibly mobilize engrammatic patterns or projections on the future.

The self can therefore once again be addressed as one of the agents and the provisional outcome of every situation. Engaged in co-creation – which does not exclude conflict – creator and created, "our perspectives slide into one another". The undifferentiated part of the intersubjective opens up to the progressive constitution of subjectivity – and thus the self – which is constantly renewed. This taking form (Gagnon, 1999) is an emerging process of contact with the immediate environment; naturally, one of the essential dimensions consists in situating in the contact with the other, but it is important not to ignore the other components of contact, the one that is established with the non-human environment (Robine, 2010).

". . . Every form has its roots in the movement that traces it: a form is nothing but recorded movement" (Bergson, 1934, p. 279).

XII

Since the self designates this ability to give form to contacts with the world, in recent years there have been more and more parallels drawn with aesthetics, allowing the discipline to extricate itself from a purely medical model. Already in the founding text, the authors stated that for their definition of the self in a situation of creative adjustment, they made reference to the creative artist and the child at play (PHG 1951, Chapter 2, §8). They draw from Otto Rank's study, *Art and Artist* (1932), which Goodman said "is beyond praise" (PHG, Chapter 11, §6 note) and on child-play. Although they do not reveal the source of that latter reference, I suppose they primarily relied on the study of G.H. Mead who himself had drawn extensively from the study of children's play to support his conception of the self (Mead, 1934).

Laura Perls (1992) liked to recall that the term "Gestalt" belonged to the vocabulary of aesthetics and, in fact, all the characteristics of a Gestalt which are listed in *Gestalt Therapy* fall within this same family.

Following this tradition, multiple studies have appeared promoting the aesthetic reference in the phenomenology of the session and the posture of the psychotherapist as much as in diagnosis, clinical settings and psychopathology (Robine, 1984, 2006a, 2006b; Miller, 2002; Alvim, 2004; Bloom, 2003, 2005; Spagnuolo Lobb, 2003, 2013; Francesetti, 2013, 2015, etc.)

We discussed the fact that when Perls and Goodman presented the self through its partial structures or functions, they mentioned that *among* the possible functions of the self, they chose three that seemed essential to enabling creative adjustment: the id-, ego- and personality-functions.

Based on contemporary developments in the theory of gestalt therapy and my own clinical experience, I attach equal importance to a fourth function: ***the aesthetic function.***

This function could bring together various forces at work in the creation of forms of contact:

- The *aesthesic* function. Aesthetics, in its original definition derived from the Greek word "aesthesis", refers to the science of sensory knowledge; it is sensitivity and sensitive individuals that make it possible to recreate meaning and existence, and generate new forms of subjectivity. What is felt – which is at the heart of the work of Erwin Straus (1970) – could take its place among the sources of experience and be differentiated from the id-function.
- The *aesthetic* function itself, which concerns the formation of forms, the reference to art that allows aesthetics to put into action and become a privileged, paradigmatic manifestation. When she describes the artist, Laura Perls formulates her description in such a way that it could equally apply to the gestalt therapist: "The main concern of the artist is certainly not the 'exercise of aesthetic transformation' of truth into beauty, but the organization of a multitude of various, disparate, incompatible experiences – which threaten the individual or society with disintegration and therefore are experienced as ugly – into a meaningful, integrated whole, a unity within which they make sense and which therefore is or may be experienced as beautiful" (Perls, 1992, p. 62).
- The *spiritual* function – which in my view cannot be based on a rational, logical way of thinking – is a form that is also rooted in the *aesthesis*: the sensitive. In certain subjects, this function seems to have a role similar to the aesthetic function in others. But perhaps this hypothesis belongs to another discussion.

This aesthetic function of the self, this formation of forms, is exercised daily in all human activity. What is emotion, then, if not a form that lets us manifest what we feel in the contact related to experienced situation and our personal history? What is a symptom if not the form that a subject constructs as a way of responding and adapting to a difficult context?

In his course at the Bauhaus, Paul Klee wrote: "The doctrine of Gestaltung deals with paths leading to the Gestalt, to the form [. . .] The word 'Gestaltung' is in direct contact with the concept [. . .] of a certain mobility" (Klee, 1956/1975).

"We seek the meaning of each form formed in the act of formation itself", as Maldiney put it (1986), summing up Prinzhorn's main contribution concerning Gestaltung (1922).

When Prinzhorn describes what he calls the movements of expression, he lists, with the vocabulary of his time, a number of components at work in the Gestaltung: the urge to play and be active, enrichment of one's surroundings, the tendency to put into order, to reproduce, the need for symbols, the need to express, to give form . . . It is easy to make connections with concepts that define the attributes and functions of the self.

The self is the formation of forms, the architect of Gestaltung, followed by the formed form, to then return to being the formation of forms . . . according to the circular modality already demonstrated by Otto Rank: "the artist not only creates his art, but also uses art in order to create" (1932/1975, p. 7).

The great psychiatrist and phenomenologist Erwin Straus (1966b) used to consider that experience is the "only authentic theme of psychology". So, he invited clinicians not to focus on mind, on nervous system, on psychic apparatus, on consciousness and so on, but on the "experiencing beings" (1966b, 249).

> The self is the organizer of contact,
> the catalyst of experience
> and the artist of life.

Context: In 2016, I edited a book entitled Self, a Polyphony of Contemporary Gestalt Therapists, *published simultaneously in French and English by Editions l'Exprimerie. The book has been translated in many countries, and the chapter presented here is my personal voice in this chorus.*

Chapter 3

A Therapy of Forms
of Experience

Many differences exist between individual gestalt therapists, as each of us has doubtless experienced. Over the years and through the diversity of contributions, the schools of thought have multiplied and the differences between them have been accentuated. These differences were first rooted in where gestalt therapy's major figures were located: the West Coast for a reference to Fritz Perls, Simkin and Claudio Naranjo; and the East Coast for Laura Perls, Paul Goodman and Isadore From. Then a middle mode between what has been defined as the theoretical rigour – or rigidity – of New York and what was described as the theatrical spontaneity of Esalen was traced by the Gestalt Institute of Cleveland and some of its pioneers, such as the Polsters. Geographical location gradually lost its importance as gestalt therapy spread beyond the borders of the United States: the different groups have sometimes been distinguished based on their key concepts: for example, contact versus awareness, as if one could exist without the other!

Over gestalt therapy's sixty-year history, other directions have developed, each one isolating or highlighting this or that brilliant intuition expressed by our founders, developing one of the nascent ideas present in the 1951 manifesto which is our foundational text, beyond its limitations and internal contradictions. The differences are now referred to under terms such as the individualistic, intrapsychic model or reference to the perspective of field and situation; the dialogical perspective; links with psychoanalytic theories of object relations or development theories; the radicalization of gestalt therapy's phenomenological position; connections with systemic and communication theories and with cognitive or neuroscience-based approaches, etc. In short, we are most likely prisoners of what Freud rightly called "the narcissism of small differences" (Freud, 1929), and it may sometimes seem as though we have drifted apart from one another, or even become somewhat foreign to each other, if not in outright conflict or trapped in a relationship of contempt or hatred.

On a number of occasions, I have asked myself a question that has concerned me for a long time: what is therapeutic in gestalt therapy? This is usually preceded by another question: is there any common ground between these diverse viewpoints?

These questions will most likely remain up for debate for a long time, which is a good thing, but I would like to make a small contribution to building a common

DOI: 10.4324/9781003515760-4

structure. I believe that what unites us – more so than what divides us – contains the main answers to these questions.

What are the implicit or explicit fundamentals at the heart of our theory and our practice? When I say "fundamentals", I am referring to those that are specific to and characteristic of gestalt therapy, rather than fundamentals that are common to multiple psychodynamic or experiential psychotherapies such as empathy, dialogue, awareness, alliance, support, transfer, etc.

1. Contact

I think I can safely say that all gestalt therapists, regardless of their convictions, place contact at the core of their theoretical work and clinical practice, although there is hardly a unanimous view of which phenomena are covered by this concept.

Contact refers to any movement between a subject and its environment: i.e. any movement of the field. It is the action that takes place at the boundary, through which the field differentiates itself into an "I" and a "not-I". It is not an experience of mutuality or reciprocity, since I can be in contact with someone without that person making any contact with me, for example by looking at or remembering the person. It is not the same as a relationship either, since "relationship" implies that the terms are related; this is not the case in contact, which is much more ephemeral.

This concept of contact sets the stage for the paradigm shift, the radical transformation brought about by Perls and Goodman. The concept of psyche was the privileged "place" of action and thus the organizer of our disciplines: psychotherapy, psychology, psychiatry, psychoanalysis, etc. But from the very first words of their foundational text, our authors resituated experience: "Experience occurs at the boundary between the organism and its environment" (Perls, Hefferline and Goodman, 1951, 1, 1).

This awareness – or intentionality, as we might say, drawing upon the work of Husserl – constructs figure/ground relations: it brings elements to the foreground, selecting extracts among the range of possibilities to make them into signifiers.

Contact is constructing meaning. Contact is constructing a form. Contact is being present in a situation. And since every situation is new, even though it may have certain similarities with previously encountered situations, each contact will involve both adaptation and creation. The forms that creative adaptation may take in a given situation are manifold, but the forms that may be taken by the interruptions, distortions, inhibitions or fixations of this creative adjustment activity are limited, and these inflections of experience are what will guide the therapeutic procedure.

2. From Feeling to Experience: The Body

The second fundamental that unites us is more difficult to explain, but I am tempted to put it into the following words: the body – and bodily feeling – is the starting point of every experience. For us, the body is awareness just as much as it is action.

I believe we would benefit from a closer reading of Merleau-Ponty in order to broaden our scope beyond a reference to Reich alone; the body is not in opposition to the mind as claimed by the model of false dichotomies denounced by Perls and Goodman. When we discuss the body, we evoke "the flesh", through which I see, move, desire and suffer. The body is the unity of being.

As a result, saying that experience is essentially the body also means that thought, emotion, feeling, artistic creation, behaviour, cognition, the unconscious, etc. are only variations of body experience.

By basing our reflections on this hypothesis, we continually strive to take up experience from its origin: bodily sensation, upstream from the games of representation that build up in successive layers until they cover up life. Experience is first and foremost made of flesh and blood.

3.   The Field and the Situation

Despite a great number of variations and implicitly or explicitly different understandings, the reference to a field perspective is also a constant among gestalt therapists. The field discussed by Perls and Goodman is not an entity; it is neither the environment nor the context. Of course every life experience is contextualized, and if this is not the case, the therapist is sure to invite the patient to contextualize his or her experience. The field proposed by Perls and Goodman is called the "organism/ environment field" because every field is the field of something or someone. There is always a structure-providing principle for a given field: the visual field of the eye; the awareness field of consciousness; the field of psychology, in which psychology is approached as the organizer of a discipline; the battlefield of a given war; etc. This case involves the organism/environment field. The use of the term "organism" rather than "person" or "subject" implies that this field cannot be defined without mentioning the body. An environment only takes on meaning through the body of the one who experiences it, in the flesh, through temporary or continued contact.

Thus the organism/environment field is specific to each organism, and cannot be a shared field.

A few years ago, I recommended that we draw on the concept of situation to expand our understanding of the field (Robine, 2001). I had noticed that the term "situation" appeared three times more often than "field" in *Gestalt Therapy*.[1] It is also easier to immediately understand the following statement: "I am the creator of the situation in which I find myself, just as I am created by this situation." This process is exactly what is described in our conception of the field.

4.   Temporality

For many of us, it would be difficult to fully understand the theoretical approach of gestalt therapy – and the practice based on it – if we did not consider the essential role it assigns to temporality in the approach to experience.

Without being too aware of it, the average person lives according to a way of thinking that hinges on two dimensions: time and space, but of these two, the spatial mode is largely dominant. We often think in terms of "above" and "below", with one type of therapy being "deeper" than another one, which is considered "superficial". The psyche is located "inside" the human being, and even our temporality is spatialized, since the past is "behind" us and the future "ahead of" us.

Although psychoanalysis has not neglected the temporal dimension of experience, particularly thanks to its focus on psychogenesis and transfer, it has certainly favoured a spatial way of thinking, which is plainly manifested by its succession of "topics". Let us recall that *topos* is Greek for "place", even though "topic" is not the same as "topological" and the principle of a psychic location is of course metaphorical.

Gestalt therapy takes this idea one step further. Without denying the spatial dimension of experience, it focuses more closely on its temporal dimension, first through its concept of the now, and more importantly with that of sequence or process.

The concept of the now is not exclusive to gestalt therapy. Otto Rank first drew attention to the importance of this approach, which made it possible to move beyond the historical-causal approach. Nonetheless, gestalt therapy was probably the most important force in popularizing the concept, occasionally leading to undesirable distortions.

Along with the now, the experience of "at the same time as" also takes on an important role in the superimposition of timelines we experience, since, in the words of Saint Augustine sixteen centuries ago, "There are three tenses or times: the present of past things, the present of present things, and the present of future things." Gestalt therapy refers to the entire span and breadth of this present.

Attached to this now is the notion of process, which goes by a number of different names: the sequence of contact, cycle, construction/destruction of gestalts, stream of consciousness, contact interruptions, etc., each of which in its own way attempts to provide an apparatus for conceptualizing movement. As far as I am aware, no other psychotherapy has devoted so much attention to the "how": how each person says what he or she says and does what he or she does. In other words, we focus more on the process than on the contents of experience. Contents stop time; processes keep it moving.

5. Form and the Formation of Forms

The last of these key concepts that I wish to address, which will occupy me a little longer, should have no trouble bringing us together. And yet – even though this is pre-eminently paradoxical – it is a concept that we use relatively little. I am referring to form. I say "paradoxical" because "form" is one of the possible translations of the German word *Gestalt*, which has no exact equivalent in other languages, at least not in any Romance language.

Since the time of Heraclitus, there has been an opposition between what flows and what remains: between the ephemeral and the stable. Since the beginnings of philosophy and of science – which for the Greeks were not separate ventures – what is stable has been given the name "form". The concept of form was then joined by other words: structure, pattern, figure, gestalt, appearance, mould, etc.

Biology, chemistry, mathematics and physics make use of this concept, as do linguistics, psychology, philosophy and aesthetics. However, for all these disciplines, beyond the unavoidable variations related to their subjects, form refers to a configuration of parts seen as a whole, and this whole is what defines the parts and renders them interdependent.

This relatively stable concept of form is joined by notions of consistency and coherence, and even of order, harmony and balance.

It took more than two millennia for the concept of form – or its equivalent, the *gestalt* – to return once again to the centre of a system of thought, albeit in a slightly different way. Gestalt psychology first examined the various factors that promote the organization of the perceptual field, before becoming gestalt theory in order to extend certain discoveries made in the realm of perception to other phenomena. With gestalt theory, the primary experience of awareness is highlighted because the perceiving form (the phenomenal pattern) is what unifies the perceived contents.

Little by little, the concept of form was separated from its visual and superficial connotations to be treated as a relative configuration of similar or related items. From this perspective, gestalt theorists argue that the interaction between the individual and the situation (dynamic field) is what determines the experience and the construction of forms, and not only the behaviour, drives, external stimuli or personality traits of a given individual.

Despite the insistence of certain authors, the concept of form is often connected to the idea of fixity and stability. Psychologists and psychotherapists are much more concerned with dynamic, temporary or metastable forms, since they are alive, than they are by static (and therefore dead) forms. This is why writers like H. Prinzhorn built their theory of the relationship between creation and pathology on the concept of *Gestaltung* and not on *gestalt*. The concept of the formation of forms is equivalent to that of *Gestaltung*.

In *Gestaltung*, emphasis is placed on the process: the movement of taking shape. Creative expression therapies focus more on the process than on the object created, while in gestalt therapy, the sequence of construction/destruction of the figure/ground relation in the present moment serves as a guide. Understanding the work of art is phenomenologically oriented toward the process as well, far from being a psychoanalytic interpretation of manifest and latent content. "We seek the meaning of each form formed in the act of formation itself", wrote Prinzhorn. The philosopher Henri Maldiney (1985; 1993; 1997) followed the same approach throughout the part of his work dedicated to art. Gestalt therapists draw on this approach to creation to guide their patients in constructing meaning based on the formation of their everyday forms of contact.

In other words, for the psychologist or psychotherapist, a form cannot be separated from its own dynamics. The scientist Philippe Quéau beautifully connects the two concepts as follows: "Forms and forces are two distinct faces of the same reality. A form is a fixed force; a force is a fluid form. Forces in action are potential forms, and vice versa."

Moreover, as we know from the aforementioned gestalt theorists, a form is given meaning both in and by the situation. Gestalt therapists would phrase it as "in contact". In an interview with Emile Noël, the epistemologist René Thom takes the example of a magnifying glass: a simple piece of glass which, when placed in a specific situation, can ignite a piece of paper by putting it in "contact" with sunlight. He also cites the example of a propeller turning in the wind which provides a stream of energy. Although these objects or forms may appear lifeless because they are immobilized, trapped within the boundaries of their own edges, might we say that they are capable of becoming metastable and "alive" once again when placed in specific situations and appropriate types of contact? A field perspective is indeed the only perspective that allows us to free ourselves from the isolationist vision of form because it connects force and form.

This conception of form is of paramount importance to psychotherapists, especially those who defined themselves as gestalt therapists, i.e. therapists of forms (meaning: that each of us has been able to give to our existence). To illustrate this perspective, I would like to briefly mention two examples of the use of a way of thinking that could be based on form: emotions and symptoms. Coincidentally, these two topics are the areas of specialization of a colleague and friend of mine based in Mexico, Myriam Muñoz. My hypothesis is that they may be united by their relation to the concept of form.

6.   An Example of the Formation of Forms: Emotion

A vast number of philosophical, phenomenological, ethological, psychological, anthropological, psychotherapeutic, sociological and other studies have been conducted on emotions, and I have no intention of calling these studies into question or contradicting them. I would just like to mention some of the issues raised by my practice of psychotherapy. What I object to among the usual theories of emotion is the assumption that emotion can be a primary phenomenon, in the sense that there is no other experience preceding it.

According to the culture, context and relational situations involved, the "emotional" experience can take different forms. Certainly, the word "emotion" comes from the Latin *ex-movere* which means "to set in motion", but it also contains the *ex* prefix that indicates the externalization of that setting in motion. In my view, what comes first is a "setting in motion" within the body, an experience that is initially only a feeling – a "pre-" experience: pre-verbal, pre-emotional, pre-significant. This is about the "vague and confused", to use Minkowski's terms. This bodily experience cannot last long without meaning or form: it is therefore given form both *in* and *by* contact, in a given situation, by "ex-" movement: exmovere, emotion, expression. I am assuming that emotion is a form produced by contact and the situation, not the production of a specific subject. Considered in this light, emotion is an indicator of the situation: it is a field phenomenon and as such, as Perls and Goodman emphasized, it reveals something about the state of the field at a given moment (i.e. of a specific organism in contact with its environment). Emotion provides information on the state of the organism confronted with the state of its environment, and thus also provides information on the characteristics of the environment in the immediacy of the situation.

Therapists often hear patients describe their pent-up anger or their unexpressed sadness. Patients can usually even locate "the emotion" within their bodies, deep down in their guts. If they are encouraged and supported in expressing this "anger", patients may utter or shout a few angry words which quickly turn into sobs. My hypothesis is that the relational and situational context, including the therapist's personality, favours one form being taken over another. As is the case in the epigenesis of the subject, a child may be explicitly asked to give another form to his feelings because the parent cannot accept the form used by the child: "Big boys don't cry!" So what does the child do in this case? He uses another form that is available and supported by his family and friends at that moment in time, such an aggressive form (since, as we know, all boys enjoy being aggressive and only girls cry!).

Yet the patient claims to experience anger that twists his stomach and that he cannot externalize. My reading is not necessarily the same as the patient's: I implicitly assume that he is having a raw bodily experience (sensation, feeling, affect) and that this experience cannot stay formless and unverbalized for very long. Based on the self's personality function – i.e. the system of self-representations drawn from prior experiences – the person uses the term "anger" for what it would probably be more accurate to describe as follows: "I feel such and such a sensation in my body and I imagine that if I were to externalize it – if I placed it in contact with the world – it would be in the form of anger!" In many cases, this may be what will happen if the situation permits it, because the subject is looking for confirmation in the representations he has of himself, so he reproduces what he knows how to do. In doing so, he locks himself inside the reproduction of a form and no longer creates contact, in relation to the elements of the situation which always involve aspects that are unknown and new. But it may also take another form . . .

As a gestalt therapist, I know that the emotions present in an encounter – both the client's and my own – represent one of the possible forms of the organization of the current experience. If it is approached as a form of experience, an emotion is an invitation to continue exploring in order to access the experience, and to consider whether this form is creation, creative adjustment and a choice from among the possible choices, rather than fixation, habit, routine or second nature. If it turns out that this form is a repetition of a fixed form, the question arises of how to re-access the possibilities of creating adjusted, creative forms.

7.   Another Example of Form: The Symptom

When placed in situations of intense difficulty, the individual is required to construct an appropriate response that incorporates the parameters of the situation. His response involves an overall configuration which includes elements that may be physical, bodily, affective, emotional, representational, motor-related, mental, relational, etc. This form, created in a given context, is a creative adjustment in that it attempts to resolve the problem as best it can using the means at hand: i.e. the materials available, affordances, codes and other resources. One of the possible forms is the symptom.

The symptom is therefore a configuration that is appropriate although sometimes uneconomical for its creator, and it has a function – even a dual function, as has been clearly shown by generations of psychologists interested in humans beyond their cognitive and behavioural components. This configuration indicates that there is a problem that it simultaneously hides *and*, through this form, tries to solve.

In a number of cases, establishing this overall configuration does actually allow the problem to be dissolved or resolved. In this case, the pattern extinguishes itself, sometimes without the subject even being aware of it.

In other cases in which attempts are made to solve the initial problem, the pattern itself may become the problem, as may be the case with obsessional rituals, addictions and many other "symptoms". The establishment of this form, which is adapted or relatively adapted to a given context, becomes obsolete through its temporal and spatial decontextualization, thereby losing most of its function. To return to the image of the propeller used by René Thom, this form was created by a given subject and adapted to provide him with energy using the force of the wind when it was necessary, but it is now being kept in a glass case that he carries around with him, regardless of where he goes and what he does.

If we accept the working hypothesis that consists in addressing the symptom as a form, thus aligning ourselves with the views of Otto Rank, who described the neurotic as a "failed artist", the therapeutic task can be approached in a perceptibly different manner (and when I say "perceptibly different", I am aware that all the "perceptible" components of this creation can thus be taken into account). This conception dates back to the early twentieth century, and it would be fruitful to extend its analysis to address symptoms as a style, not only as a disease.[2]

The symptom is a form: one which has been adapted and is appropriate to a situation, a context and/or a relational system – a form of contact. It is most definitely an inflected form, suffering and generating suffering, because it is often full of clumsy missteps. This form externalizes, expresses and says something to someone. It is there for a reason, even if it is not always easy to understand its origin, its choice, its meaning, its function, its grammar or its lexicon. If the form's adjustment characteristics are obsolete, the therapeutic task can be designed around the construction of new forms, with the destruction of fixed forms in favour of fluid, metastable forms which to the fullest extent possible should be more economical, better suited to the situation and more efficient in their functioning. Incidentally, this is one reason why many psychotherapists – or many gestalt therapists, at least – attach so much importance to the development of creative processes, and to this end, as part of the healing process, implement the use of artistic mediators: they provide a training ground or test site for the creation of forms of existence.

8.   Conclusion: Psychotherapy as an Aesthetic

Therapists who dare to place the concept of form at the centre of their approach to human experience thereby remove the concept of disease from its position as the essential paradigm. Their type of psychotherapy is characterized not only by a scientific approach[3] but first and foremost by an aesthetic approach, i.e. one that is anchored in a philosophical approach based on the sensitive qualities of form. Health is thus addressed as the ability to create forms that are adapted to situations, and pathology as the loss of this potential which leads to reliance on fixed forms which are inadequate or obsolete – scribbling. The concept of form also brings together all the fundamentals outlined earlier. As Bergson observed, "every form has its roots in a movement that traces it: a form is nothing but recorded movement" (Bergson, 1934, p. 279).

This certainly does not come with the corollary that psychotherapists have to define or identify themselves as artists, contrary to the claims of some in an attempt to justify their refusal to acquire the techniques and knowledge required for such an exercise. While working with a therapist, the patient is able to become a kind of artist – a creator of his or her existence: that is to say, forms that are flexible, significant, limited, coherent, articulate, adjusted, creative and consistent. In the words of Isadore From, a member of the group that founded gestalt therapy, the goal of psychotherapy is to help clients "transform their speech into poetry and their walk into dance" – work that involves the formation of forms.

Context: I have a particular affection for this essay: it's the text of the closing address of the 11th International Conference for Gestalt Therapy, held in Madrid in 2009, which brought together some 1,000 professionals, mostly from so-called "Latin" countries. The organizers knew we all were sitting on a powder keg, as differences in references and approaches diverged from country to country, and sometimes even within the same country, and could take on very conflicting forms, whether in Latin America or Europe. Even though I'm not opposed to conflictual expression, which can be creative, I wanted to conclude our meeting by highlighting what brought us together, despite our sometimes very different vocabulary, and which at the same time could constitute the origi-nality of gestalt therapy, over and above the ingredients common to all psycho-dynamic and/or relational approaches.

Notes

1 339 times for "situation" in the French translation, versus 131 for "field" (*champ*).
2 See, for example, Steiner and Moralès (1997).
3 The current trend, with the complicity of the public authorities, encourages the so-called "scientific" approach to psychotherapy. It has only succeeded in creating a temporar-ily profitable illusion; a wide range of studies have clearly shown that the supposedly scientific nature of this approach was nothing but an illusion: the "scientistic" mask of corporatist lobbying.

Chapter 4

Contact, at the Source of Experience

Fore

Contact is the most important organizing concept of gestalt therapy theory. *Contact* refers to all the movements of a given organism and its environment; that is, all the field movements. Contact is therefore the phenomenon that precedes any organization of experience: pre-Oedipal, pre-object, pre-conscious pre-representation, pre-emotional, pre-psychic . . . Becoming sedimented in a "psyche", experience was and will be again contact, for it is in and through contact that the psyche will *ex*-ist and preside over future experiences. The *pre* is both genesis and structure.

This concept originates and confirms the shift of paradigm, the radical change brought and organized by Perls and Goodman with the creation of gestalt therapy. Before them, the psyche was the lens and object privileged by the "psy"s *psy*chotherapy, *psy*chology, *psy*chiatry, *psy*choanalysis . . . However, since the first words of their founding text, our authors have relocated experience because experience occurs at the boundary between the organism and its environment, one of the fundamental topics suggested by Perls and Goodman. Contacting and being contacted are the actions operating at the boundary and thanks to which the field differentiates into an I and a not-I.

This concept, doubtlessly because of its apparent simplicity and common usage, became increasingly distorted, little or not all differentiated from that of relationship. It has been used for an ethics of dialog, an ideology of relationship, or for inscribing gestalt therapy in the premier ranks of "relational psychotherapies".

Certainly, as much research confirms, an important factor, essential even, that determines the success of a psychotherapy, whatever that may be, resides within the quality of the relationship created between the therapist and the client, as well as with the quality of their therapeutic alliance. But gestalt therapy is *not primarily* centred on the quality of the relationship between therapist and patient for that is not an end in itself but the means. It is the means of exploring, working and transforming as much as necessary the qualities of an individual's relationship with what is "other" and his environment, human and non-human.

DOI: 10.4324/9781003515760-5

With

Certainly, if a red surface and a blue surface are in contact, they do not create a violet line when they are united, even if this is hallucinated through an illusion of perception, as shown by Brentano. Contact is not a mutual or reciprocal experience because we can be in contact with someone or something, for instance by gaze or by memory, without this person or object being in the least bit of contact with us. The very definition of reciprocity implies the equal exertion of an action by the first to the second as by the second to the first.

However *con*-tact implies *with*. Touch with. It is definitely this "with" that generates shifts in meaning, there being so many possibilities of being "with". "I am so *with* this film I saw last week . . .", "I'll go for a ride *with* my car", "I am and will be *with* you in this difficult time . . .", "I'd love to live *with* you . . ." The etymological reference to tactility increases ambiguity because touching is the only one of the five senses that implies reciprocity: I can see you without being seen, hear you without being heard . . . I cannot touch you without being touched. When I touch a keyboard I am simultaneously touched by it, but this does not at all refer to a lived *experience*, a fundamental aspect when the contact is interhuman. I experience touching a keyboard, but the keyboard does not *live* this experience with me. Contact is therefore also a form of consciousness, a "knowing with."

If I establish physical contact with someone, like pinching their arm, their probably painful experience with this contact will be fundamentally different from the one I lived through. Even if contact is an act that puts into play a "with" and a "being", the lived experience cannot be considered the same because "with" does not mean "sameness". On the contrary, in this example, it allows differentiation.

All contact implies placement being in the presence of otherness, of *two*. Maybe it is better said as: *experienced as* two. When some therapists suggest to their clients to "get in contact with their feelings", it shows that these therapists, in their anthropology or their *weltanschauung* (world view), consider feelings as separate and distinct from the self, and they transmit this implicit notion to their client. It is paradoxical for those who mean to unite experience into a single Gestalt!

Sometimes it may indeed make sense for a patient to express themselves in this way, like when parts of their own body are experienced as strange or foreign. Perls and Goodman cite the case in which a pain is localized in a body part and not experienced as "me", but as something that happened to me, as if it came from "outside" . . . and that does not belong to me.

Sometimes the therapist's language can help the client reappropriate their experience as well as it can create, amplify, or support the separation or splitting.

Contact as Awareness

For Perls and Goodman, awareness is characterized by contact, by sensing, by excitement and by Gestalt formation. The connection between awareness and contact was established with the introduction of *gestalt therapy* when they affirm that "contact as such is possible without awareness, but for awareness contact is indispensible". I am in contact with the ground, with the seat on which I sit, with the air that I breathe. These forms of contact are sometimes called "physiological" or "physical" and are opposed to "psychological" forms that imply consciousness – even if implicit – and the construction of a figure. However, the patterns of this "physiological" contact (I maintain this mediocre terminology for lack of a more satisfying one) are not in opposition to the "physiological" modalities. There really and truly is a continuation from one to the other: my manner of being in contact with the ground is related by analogy to my roots; my manner of breathing is coherent with my other exchange modalities of taking and giving with the environment. These apparently distinct planes can be legitimately approached as *consistency* of experience. They should be considered as a continuity within the breadth of experience and not as a distinct modality. J.-P. Sartre wrote:

> Thus the connection between the world and awareness is one of contact. The world exists for the awareness in so far as the world is concretely and singularly what the awareness is not. The awareness touches the world since its partial neutralization can establish exteriority without distance between them. The world is neither subjective nor objective: it is the 'it-self' that invades and contacts the awareness, just as the awareness passes the world in its nothingness.
>
> (1995, p. 400ff.)

Non-awareness and non-contact are called *confluence* in gestalt therapy. This non-awareness consists of habits and knowledge, of facts gathered throughout experience and through introjects. Certain confluent experiences remain potentially contactable. For example, it is possible to question the legitimacy of a spontaneously used word; that is, to bring the word into figural while I am in a relationship of confluence with my mother language. Other experiences are harder to contact because of repression or other modes of fixation.

A Figure/Ground Relation

"Contact [. . .] is the forming of a figure of interest against a ground or context of the organism/environment field" (PHG, 1951–2001, p. 54). This awareness, or, relying on the works of Brentano and then Husserl, this *intentionality*, builds figure/ground relationships. It brings to the foreground and selects within the field of possibilities excerpts that can become significant.

Contact, therefore, aims and builds meaning. *Contacting* is building a form. "Form is where organism and its milieu meet", Weizsäcker wrote already in 1940 and, as a consequence, Maldiney (1990b) was able to advance that the formation of forms creates existence.

To be certain of using the concept of contact in a coherent manner, it would be preferable to systematically add to the word "contact" not just "with whom or with what" but "through which modalities".

Regarding the question "with whom or what?", I would readily suggest to come back to the introduction of Perls, Hefferline and Goodman's book. "The crucial question is: with what is one in contact? The spectator of a modern painting may believe that he is in contact with the picture while he is actually in contact with the art critic of his favorite journal" (PHG, 1951–2001, p. 39). This raises, among others, the question of transference: beyond perceptual and sensorial contact, with whom is my client in contact?

Touching, seeing, hearing . . . are regular modes of contact, but so are remembering, fantasizing, thinking, being excited, singing, writing, dreaming, being moved and so on. I can contact a friend by looking at him, hearing him, telephoning him, touching him, going to see him, remembering him, anticipating him, imagining him . . .

We can use as a basis the principle of noetic-noematic variations as elaborated by Husserl regarding consciousness to apply to contact. When I establish contact with someone, like a patient, I contact this person and this person contacts me. We do not have the same contact "object", the same contents or even the same objective. (This is the noematic aspect of experience: the other as *noema*.)

"Thinking", "loving", "hating", "imagining" . . . they are all verbs for what the mind does. Walking, breathing, feeling, thinking, hearing, going to, fantasizing, dreaming . . . are contacting types or modalities (noesis). With the same "object" (the "other", for example), I can have different types of contact: touching, hearing, looking, remembering him/her, feeling, projecting, cautioning, thinking of him/her, loving him/her . . .

But the contacting modalities can be united around two axes, two essential movements: going towards or distancing. Or, in other words, integrating or differentiating; fusing or separating; linking or unlinking; belonging or diverging . . . "(Contact) leads to touching and uniting [. . .]. The stakes of contact and its risks will be as much about leading to an encounter where a separation occurred as being able to separate from an integral union right down to the fusion", wrote Lekeuche (1990, p. 34). It is also the double movement of contact introduced in the bipartition brought by Imre Hermann in "clinging" and "going out to search". This will be extended by Balint in his description of "ocnophile" types (to cling, to hang on) and "philobate" (going out to search).

Inflexions of Contacting

In an interview with E. Glassheim (1973), Paul Goodman answered one of his questions, ". . . the soul is wherever the action is, that's where the soul is, where the action is". And since each situation is new, even if it has similarities to previous encounters, each contact will be at the time adjustment and creation. The forms that can entail creative adaptation within a given situation are many, but the forms that can take on the interruptions, distortions, inhibitions, and fixations of this creative adjustment are limited. It is precisely towards these "inflexions" of experience that the therapeutic act will be focused.

Rather than using the phrase "interruptions of contact", a concept that generates ambiguities, I proposed in 1997 (Robine, 1997a, p. 125), following Binswanger's tradition, the use of the term "inflexion". This term, borrowed from linguistics, refers to the ensemble of modifications of a word to express different grammatical categories such as a tense, a grammatical voice, gender and so on. Transposed to the topic that interests us, the modality variations, the deformations and other fluctuations in contacting are thus not subject to the opprobrium that the idea of interruption can bring. However, when Perls et al. discuss interruptions of contact, it is important to keep in mind that they believe that "the on-goingness of the process will not be lost". They believe that, in the sequence of contacting, creativity can be interrupted by certain modalities and that therefore contact can eventually be carried on within routines or acted by a reduced self (i.e. losses of ego-functions of the self).

If contact accompanies each movement between a subject and its environment, which is to say all movement OF THE field, contact is an act, not a result. It is therefore more relevant to speak of *contacting* because actions are better expressed through verbs than nouns. Gestalt therapy promotes a culture of verbs over that of nouns, adjectives or adverbs.

When I listen to a patient, it is the verbs of his narrative that I most eagerly listen to. This is because they describe the processes, actions and contacting according to modalities that can often be considered his experiences as such, if not, sometimes, as a metaphor or metonym of his experience.

About Contact at the Contact-Boundary

Beautifully expressed by Eugen Fink (1952, pp. 70–71), "To appear means, for a singular essence or being, its coming into the open, its advent between sky and earth, in space-interval and time-interval." The concept of contact-boundary is a direct consequence of contact and represents a specific practical interest. Nonetheless, there is often confusion between "contact-boundary" and "boundary" or "boundaries" in the use of this concept that resembles that of, for example, structural family therapy: limits, contours. This is the case of the different boundaries Erv and Miriam Polster described, which have little connection to Perls' and Goodman's concept of contact-boundary, which can cause much confusion. "Contact-boundary" is a sort of epistemological abstraction, such as with "self". There is no good reason to reify or to transform an experience into an object and thereby justify speaking of "one's" contact-boundary as could be said of actual boundaries.

When teaching this concept, I sometimes use an analogy drawn from the way the famous philosopher Merleau-Ponty taught his own difficult concepts. Most of the time, I am not aware of my hand because I do not feel any specific sensation there. When I lay my hand on an object or on somebody's shoulder, through the same act I feel my hand and I feel the object or the other. Touching this object gives it existence in my tactile experience and, through the same operation, it gives sensations, thus existence, to my hand. It's contact that simultaneously gives existence to the other and to me and which, by the same token, differentiates one from the other. The same operation, the same act, separates and joins. Contact creates a boundary and boundary creates contact as well. Without contact, there is no differentiation; without differentiation, there is no contact, thus no experience.

(Robine, 2007)

Contact is touch touching something, sight is neither the eye nor the object but the oval of vision. It thus links the eyes with the world that is seen. At work is a process similar to that shown by Husserl when he said that there is no "consciousness" but only the "consciousness of" something.

An experience can seem to be intrapsychic when it actually is a contact-boundary event. An event continues because we are always engaged in one contact or other.

This has many consequences for psychotherapy. Every client describes the majority of their experiences as an intrapsychic suffering: shame, guilt, hatred, neglect, rejection, anger, conflict, and so on. These experiences should be considered as contact experiences. By considering them not as solipsistic phenomena but as contact-boundary phenomena, it changes the perspective and has an extremely powerful therapeutic impact. If "the contact-boundary is the organ of awareness" (Robine, 2007, p. 85), then contact-boundary, as experience, is the prime "location" where the therapist and client should work together.

Post

After some sixty years of gestalt therapy, which has been marked by the introduction of "contact as first experience" that brought multiple practical and methodological consequences, it is surprising that the gestalt community should be little interested in refining, enriching and differentiating this concept. It was an important concept in the works of the Hungarian School of Psychoanalysis (Hermann and Balint, whom have already been mentioned, as well as Spitz, Mahler, and especially Szondi, whose work was continued by Jacques Schotte). This concept would today benefit from the enrichment through the works of Todorov; Bin Kimura's concept of aïda; Winnicott's concept of betweeness; Lacan and other psychoanalysts; and Merleau-Ponty's and Maldiney's works . . . It is also important to articulate the concept of contact within the context of relationships, particularly of therapeutic relations, which are non-reducible to contact, transference, projective identification, interaction, communication, dialogue or intersubjectivity.

But if we must investigate "action-passion" and "combination," we must also investigate 'contact.' For action and passion (in the proper sense of the terms) can only occur between things which are such as to touch one another; nor can things enter into combination at all unless they have come into a certain kind of contact. Hence we must give a definite account of these three things—of "contact," "combination," and "acting."

(Aristotle, 1866, I, ch. 6, §4)

Context: *The concept of contact is undoubtedly the one on which, in my eyes, the whole theoretical, practical and clinical edifice of gestalt therapy rests. It was with this concept that I made my first attempts at gestalt-therapy writing around 1979–80, and it's the one I keep coming back to, to better understand the scope of this paradigm, so commonplace and so original at the same time. This new essay was to have two readers: the* Cahiers de Gestalt-thérapie, *which in 2010 in France devoted its issue no. 25 to the theme of "Contacter", and the Brazilian online magazine* Aw@re, *now defunct, which in its issue 2011, no. 2 wanted to open up a major debate on this theme and submitted my essay to the in-depth comments of Dan Bloom, from the New York Institute for Gestalt Therapy, and Selma Ciornai and Lilian Frazão, from two Brazilian Gestalt Institutes.*

Chapter 5

Does the Now Have a Future?

To begin this reflection on the now, I would like to mention a few memories of experiences that have represented question marks – if not breaks – in my conception of time.

In the late sixties, I had finished my undergraduate studies in psychology and was working on completing a master's degree in psychopathology.

My master's thesis involved a psychodrama group of children that I had been following over a period of two or three years. I had not yet been through any personal therapy, other than the psychodrama group therapy I was involved in at the time. There were aspects of the way this group (and the children in it) functioned that I didn't understand, despite the regular supervisory work I was doing; I didn't understand some of the working hypotheses on a theoretical level, and one day I talked about it with my research director, who was quite a well-known psychoanalyst, and he told me, "There's one thing that you haven't yet grasped: the Freudian unconscious is timeless; the unconscious has no conception of time." This statement seemed quite mysterious at the time, and the professor did not provide any further hints as to what it might mean. I found myself in a similar situation to what I encountered later with some of Goodman's proposals: the speaker makes a statement and gives us hardly any clues to understand his point. It took me a number of years of clinical practice to understand it through my own psychoanalysis, based on personal experience as much as clinical experience, and to illustrate it using the example of a dream – whether from a Gestalt perspective or a psychoanalytic one, moreover. In a dream we may find people we met yesterday, people from our childhood, strangers, people we know well, prehistoric processes, current processes, expectations and so on, all coexisting. All these elements operate in a mode that Freud called *condensation*: they are all condensed, and there is no specific temporality. Since the unconscious has no conception of time, ingredients from yesterday have the same status as elements from twenty years ago; they all coexist in the experience of a dream. Time is condensed in a dream, and the same is true for the present moment. One might say that there is no time in the present moment either, because the present, the past and the future are intimately mixed and condensed – it is thick, full of strata: coexisting, overlapping or even interwoven layers. The present moment contains everything.

DOI: 10.4324/9781003515760-6

Some gestalt therapists (such as Frank Staemmler and Erving Polster) have challenged this "terrorism of the now" in articles such as Polster's "Imprisoned in the present" or other examples along these lines. For my part, I believe that we are imprisoned in the present because yesterday no longer exists and the future does not yet exist. However, that does not mean we should refuse to talk about the past or the future; instead, we therapists should be aware that things are happening now, and that this has meaning in relation to the now. This is how I think we should understand both Staemmler and Polster. I will return to this later on.

Moreover (and this is the second powerful experience that I wanted to mention), I remember having a discussion with Erving Polster about what Goodman had taught him and what had stuck with him from his teachings, and the first thing he said to me was essentially that Goodman had given him a different conception of time: one that changed his life. He briefly explained his conception of time, which led me to read *Gestalt Therapy* for the umpteenth time in order to dis-cover the confirmation of this implicit conception of time. According to this conception, time is not only linear. In other words, in the implicit conception of time that more or less all of us have without even being aware of it, being fifty years old means no longer being forty years old, no longer being thirty years old, no longer being twenty years old, no longer being ten years old, no longer being five years old, no longer being one year old, no longer being three months old, etc. Childrearing is also organized around this principle, with parents saying to their children, "Listen to me! You aren't five years old anymore!" I myself often find myself noticing that I am no longer twenty years old when I see certain types of physical exertion that I have a hard time doing.

However, Goodman's conception of temporality is quite different since it is implicitly based on the idea that being sixty years old means being fifty years old AND twenty years old AND ten years old AND two years old AND six months old, and so on, all at the same time. It is another kind of condensation, and one might imagine it also meaning that being sixty years old would also mean being seventy years old AND eighty years old . . . but Polster did not mention that in his understanding of Goodman's ideas.

For me, meditating on this idea for several weeks after my interview with Polster changed a lot. It gave me a freedom and a flexibility that provides me with a great deal of opportunities, such as playing like a child and not worrying about the idea that it's not for people my age; being able to play and contact my grandchildren or my friends' children, not by acting *as if* I were three years old, but by *being* there as my own *current* three-year-old self. Simply engaging with this mode of looking at the world gave me a great deal of freedom.

There's a word I've used in some of the articles I've written, which I very much like and would like to have the chance to use again: the word "consistency", which Simondon uses quite frequently. In the present moment, there is this "consistency". Being sixty years old *consists* of being fifty years old, thirty years old, etc. But when we talk about the "consistency" of a vegetable soup or a theory, we are saying that these things have a certain thickness; we are referring to the material they contain. I think this concept of consistency is interesting in our context.

Goodman's idea of temporality as accumulation and consistency led me to think a little differently about the theory of the sequence of contact, process and flow. Something bothered me when I used this sequence of contact in follow-up work and to dissect my own work. According to our teaching, this sequence is traditionally represented as a linear curve, but when I looked at my work in a session, I didn't see myself progressing linearly but rather taking certain steps forward and other steps backward, in something that was not as linear as what this famous curve supposedly offered. By drawing on Goodman's underlying conception of time, we might instead represent this curve as a kind of stack, with the idea that at every moment of the process, in its entire breadth, we can find this consistency. Let's take a concrete example: my patient and I are in the contact phase. He tries something; you may recall that the contact phase consists of going towards the environment and identifying/alienating ("This concerns me; this doesn't interest me; I'll keep this as a figure; I'll place that in the background", etc.). In this phase, I go towards the "object" to meet it. At the beginning of this meeting between me and the object that I identify and which seems to correspond to what I am looking for, I may realize that ultimately this may not be what I want. What do I do then? I refine the contours of my desire, my need, my appetite, my drive and my going-towards, and my environment may also invite or compel me towards it. In other words, I find myself back in the pre-contact phase. This is what Goodman (who may have borrowed the idea from Isadore From) meant when he said that pre-contact and the other phases of the sequence are both *moments* of the experience and *modes* of experience. Certain pre-contact phases may be nothing more than *pre-contact*: they will never be followed by contact and thus remain experiences of pre-contact, which does not however mean that we need to consider them unfinished situations. When I see someone go by, I establish a sort of pre-contact by looking at the person I see there, and the experience does not go any further. In this way, pre-contact can be both a *mode* and a *moment*.

With the example I just used, the attempt to make contact brings me back to the refinement of my desire, my need and my appetite, and in this mode of representation it does not have to be considered a step backward (and this is where I was not satisfied). There is no step backward! This would justify the use of the concept of regression. As we know, Freud developed three types of regression: temporal regression (retreating backward in time), topical regression (retreating from a given topical modality to an earlier, less advanced topical modality), and formal regression. In my opinion, temporal regression does not make much sense, even on a symbolic level. What is referred to as regression might often be just as well seen as progression, since it may represent another way forward, but we'll save that for another debate! When we are in the contact phase, there is no turning back; in this contacting phase – the thickness or consistency of making contact – pre-contact work continues.

As a result of the thickness of the moment, everything is contained in the present.

This makes me think of St Augustine's concept of time, which he developed in the fourth and fifth century CE. He said that there are three tenses or times: the present of past things, the present of present things, and the present of future things. There is no past or future: only the present. Remembering thus takes place in the present of past things. One hypothesis states that something in the present moment causes a certain memory and not another to appear *now*. The *structure* of the present moment – of the current experience – is what causes a specific memory to appear and superimpose itself on the experience of the present moment.

Let's try to understand what I call the "structure" of the current experience.

If I say a word or phrase – for example, "to be" – each of you have associations that will immediately spring to your mind. Some people will think of personal qualities, such as being handsome or boring; others will think of the idea of being itself, perhaps as opposed to doing, or of existing in this world. Each and every listener will associate a particular, specific way of being with the words "to be".

If I am more specific and say "to be or not", I have already limited your experience, and certain specific memories and images are associated and engaged. Do I exist or not? How do I know? Or maybe you remember things your philosophy teacher talked about in high school.

But if I instead say "to be or not to be", what happens? There is a particular structure and a specific process in my sentence construction that will probably conjure up a specific, shared memory in nearly every English-speaking person who hears it: the famous line in Shakespeare's play *Hamlet*. It is a particular *structure of experience*. My hypothesis is as follows: our memory and the calling forth of unfinished situations, childhood experiences and other memories in the present moment functions in a way that is based much more on *processes* than on *content*.

"To be (or not)" involves quite a different syntactic process than "to be or not to be", in the context of our shared history. If I say the latter, you most likely cannot help but think of the line in *Hamlet*.

I believe that this is how the present moment functions. The present moment, with its entire thickness, operates based on engaged processes. I consider this another reason to insist on paying attention to verbs when we listen to our patients. Verbs are where actions and contact are found. Contact, which we work on in gestalt therapy, is always an action. There is no contact without action. *No* contact can exist without action. Contact requires us to at the very least look towards or listen to something or someone; as a result, there is always some motor function involved in contact. In our language, this motor function is always expressed by verbs because verbs describe action. When I say "chair", there is no action. When I say "sitting in a chair", there is or has been an action. I listen to actions; I can isolate verbs and imagine (in hypothetical terms, of course) the action my patient is describing; I can decontextualize and recontextualize it because in the thickness and consistency of the moment, this action is what is important: the *structure of the process of the experience*, not the content. In an article I once wrote, I took the example of a patient who told me he'd dreamed he was writing and dropped his pen. On the surface, it sounds like a very uninteresting dream. But the action encapsulated in the verb is "dropped"! "Are you perhaps trying to tell me that you feel like I've dropped you or let you down?" "Are you perhaps trying to tell me that you want to drop therapy?" (Of course I wouldn't say this so abruptly.) In the present moment, an action is condensed with other actions, memories, plans, etc.

A metaphor that has been widely used to characterize gestalt therapy's approach is that of a hologram: the holographic approach as a way of thinking. A hologram, as you probably know, is a kind of picture that produces a three-dimensional image. Let's compare this with a product of a traditional film camera, such as a slide, even though these days slides and slide projectors are hardly used anymore. A slide is a transparent photo: you send a beam of light through the image and the projector's lenses project a larger version of this image on your wall. The 24x36mm landscape in the photo is reproduced identically but much larger on the wall in front of you. If I cover part of the source picture, thus sending light through only part of the slide, only the equivalent portion will be blown up on my wall. With a hologram, the result is completely different: even if I send a beam of light through only a small portion of the image, I'll still have the whole picture projected on the wall. In other words, each point of the "photo" contains the whole image. Of course, the picture projected on the wall will be clearer if light is shone through a larger portion of the source photo. Nevertheless, each point of the "slide" contains the entire photo.

This metaphor is sometimes used to illustrate gestalt therapy's approach, namely the fact that the whole is contained within each of its "elements", a metonym for experience.

We might say, as Perls and others have done, that everything is in the present moment. The problem of course lies in knowing how to see it, decode it and understand it. You have probably experienced this as a patient and perhaps even as a therapist: when you dissect and unfold the present moment, you are able to understand something about its history and origins. At times, this may seem like a magic trick to the patient, who hears you formulating hypotheses about his or her past based on the present moment!

Nevertheless, it is also true that while everything is in the present moment, at the same time *not* everything is in the present moment. For example, when I listen to music, if I isolate a note, I do not have the entire symphony, and the note itself only has meaning and impact because it has a before and an after. I have a short-term memory of the musical phrase and the note that I am listening to, which changes from one moment to the next and is part of a process in flux; the outline of this flux is what makes sense.

A question thus arises for the therapist: which end of the present moment am I going to start with? As soon as I start trying to grasp it, it has already disappeared. This is the source of a number of confusions, as we can see for example in Daniel Stern's most recent book, *The Present Moment in Psychotherapy and Everyday Life*, which many gestalt therapists swear by. Thanks to this book, psychoanalysis discovered the present moment! It even timed the length of this moment: it lasts about 7 seconds! We clearly do not all have the same understanding of what "the present moment" means. It is true that the present moment is part of a process: that there is a before and an after. If I represent it on an axis as the arrow of time, a certain point on the arrow represents the present moment and, as in music, it has a before and an after. How can I observe it? I can either look in the rear-view mirror or look towards the "next". These are two different approaches; neither one is more right or more wrong than the other. In what psychoanalysts call transfer, based on what is happening in the present moment between the psychoanalyst and the patient, the therapy will tend to be oriented towards trying to return to primary patterns such as the Father–Child or Mother–Child relational matrix and how we learned to build relationships according to our early methods, all based on the assumption that what is here now is an attempt to replicate these childhood patterns. This means that this approach based on the transfer hypothesis is deeply rooted in exploring the relation between the present and the past. To put it simply, according to the different schools of psychoanalysis two fundamental orientations are possible: those who use the present to better understand the past, and those who use the past to better understand the present. It's a choice that makes sense. If you look at your present moment, your presence here is the result of a history: a path; perhaps it was your therapy that sparked your desire to become a therapist, and perhaps this dream of being a therapist goes back your childhood, since you may already have been full of symptoms – perhaps you were already your family's therapist! The present moment may be seen as the outcome of the past: the result of a long history. Of course, if I were only meant to look at the present, your presence here would not make much sense; if there were nothing behind and nothing ahead, or if you knew you were going to die in a matter of minutes, you might have more interesting things to do than listen to me. The present moment does not make sense in isolation. We can also understand the present moment in terms of a future: your plan to become a therapist or a better therapist, or to be part of a network of colleagues you enjoy working with. In other words, your future is also what gives meaning to your present moment. It is a choice: another methodological choice. One is no truer than the other; it is a professional orientation choice.

At the Gestalt Therapy General Convention, Daniel Stern said something that made me jump: "If the present couldn't change the past, psychotherapy wouldn't be worth doing." We can understand what he meant, but his statement represents a serious epistemological shift because psychotherapy has never changed the past! What exists is only the present of past things (cf. St Augustine), and what we might be able to change is the present representation we have of our past. We can change the impact of the past on the present moment. To plagiarize and tweak Polster's formula, I would say we should stop being "trapped in the past".

What I believe is that for some patients, it is quite useful to explore their personal history, their narrative and the stories they tell. "My past" is clearly a story I like to tell myself. It doesn't necessarily match how things actually happened, but that's why I need to tell myself the story: a "rhetorical attitude", as Goodman would say. It is therefore a fiction, as is my identity. I absolutely need these elements because they are points of support, but they are fictional, even though this fiction may have its relevance, effectiveness and usefulness.

My choice is the following: if we are in a therapeutic perspective, what we can change is what comes next. We can't change the past but we can orient the *next*. According to Goodman's "Here-now-next" formulation, "here" refers to space, "now" refers to time, and "next" involves both time AND space; it designates what is temporally and spatially close to us.

My working hypothesis and my suggestion would therefore be to focus our approach preferably on the "now and next": to consider each moment as containing tension to propel us towards the following moment. Each moment contains a plan.

Speaking of this, I would like to make a slight detour towards Husserl, one of the founders of phenomenology. There can be no temporality without time-consciousness. Husserl worked extensively on consciousness. He taught us something simple: that "consciousness" does not exist as such. What exists is "consciousness of –": "of" something; there is no consciousness without an object of consciousness, just as a memory is always a memory OF something. A memory without content is not a memory. This consciousness, which is consciousness of something, therefore has a target; this is what he called the intentionality of consciousness. That's the philosophical component. I myself, as a psychotherapist, psychologist or otherwise, also believe that this target is not neutral. What underpins it? Kurt Lewin, for example, among others, argued that this target was oriented by need, or more accurately – and I like this way of describing it – rather than the concept of need, he preferred to use the term "pseudo-need", since we are always a little "off". This is also what we say about the id. As a result, needs or pseudo-needs are what structure our intentionality: they provide us with targets. If "you" are what I'm looking at in this moment, for the moment I don't know anything about it but if we made the effort to unfold the encounter, we would see that my consciousness is drawn there because there is a target, and this target is supported by a plan, by intentionality, or by something implicit. Our work as therapists may be to reveal this target and this intentionality, which will only materialize through an extract or a portion of this potential. If I look at you, my regard involves a vague, confused intentionality that may materialize in the form of meeting for drinks, for example, but it could also take many other forms, including spending our lives together! Initially, the spectrum is very broad, but when we reach the register of intention, the spectrum gradually narrows, becoming deliberate, chosen and limited. A therapist's job is perhaps to guide the return to intentionality, the status of intentionality, and what is raw and felt, since this is related to intentionality. My working hypothesis is that there is always some intentionality; there is always some id growing in every situation, and the id always pushes towards the next, never towards the past, of course. Even though it is sometimes said that the patient wants to go backwards or that he closes himself off by repeating the past, the id always pushes towards the next, and when I discuss my present moment, we may understand the present moment as containing the next. If I say "I'm hungry", I describe my present moment but I also implicitly say what I want to come next. I do not explicitly describe the next; I describe my bodily condition. Of course, this does not mean that the therapist needs to wait to hear this implicit element in order to respond to it. When a patient says "I am sad", he isn't only saying "I'm sad"; folded up in this statement, he is also describing a desire and a direction of meaning, but I don't know what it is and neither does he. It is up to us to unfold it together.

My work as a therapist thus consists of helping my patient support the present moment so that he orients himself more willingly towards the next than towards the past.

If I go towards the past, I will encourage the action of the personality function: the reproduction of the same.

In the present moment, there is everything and there is novelty present at every moment.

I'd like to say a few words about the issue of therapist disclosure because it is a topic that has a lot to do with the question of the now.

Many gestalt therapists consider it very important to self-disclose: to reveal things about themselves. I think that even a psychotherapist who only utters one word every six months practises a form of self-disclosure, as paradoxical as that may seem: he reveals something about his constipation (*laughs*). I use the image of constipation because I'm reminded of a patient in the 1940s who said to Moreno, the founder of psychodrama, "Master, if I have to die, I'd rather die of diarrhoea with you than of constipation with Freud." According to the theory of communication developed by Watzlawick et al., "One cannot not communicate." I say something about myself by remaining silent, and we should never assume that just because we say nothing we are completely silent. For this reason, psychotherapists are not just blank screens; whether they like it or not, they are not neutral. The patient reacts to silence; his speech is a *reaction* to their verbal silence.

The gestalt therapist may employ a certain level of self-disclosure, but what I often notice in supervision and direct observation is that this disclosure is often very cumbersome for the patient. When you are a beginner, it is easy to imagine that by talking about yourself, you will provide support to the patient. I believe it can sometimes be useful, but it can also be invasive and intrusive, and more importantly it can deprive the patient of something: it robs him of the chance to disclose his own experience.

This creates a pseudo-closeness that may be completely demagogic. It's not about describing my life or my relationship with my grandmother. On the other hand, the therapist's disclosure may play a fundamental part in the here and now. Being in the here and now means I can say something about my now, insofar as my now is jointly constructed by our encounter. If I am sad now, this sadness is a product of our encounter (meaning it is created or activated by our encounter); if I am angry now, this anger is a product of our encounter. Obviously, this sadness or anger may also have something to do with my past and my personal history, since what the patient is telling me reactivates the thickness of my experience. However, this does not concern the patient and, anyway, even if this sadness has something to do with my personal history, the feeling is awakened and activated by our meeting now. Describing what I'm feeling helps to clarify the process that is taking place here and now, between you and me.

If I'm worried, at some point, this worry is a product of the session. I think it's interesting to consider that in principle this worry is not my own: to methodologically position it in the realm of the undifferentiated. This is the initial non-differentiation of the session: not "We are the same" but rather the position of uncertainty from which we began. If I walk towards a patient and she says, "I'm anxious when I see you approaching me", the therapist may be tempted to explore her anxiety: "What does this remind you of? What is your anxiety like? How do you feel it in your body?" and so on. This of course implies that the anxiety belongs to you! I came towards you with kindness, tenderness and affection; there's no way this anxiety could be mine in any way! In reality, I may not be aware of how I may be perceived by the patient, or by anyone else, for that matter. The patient may perceive things that I can't: something about me that may be much more threatening than I can imagine. This means that while the patient's anxiety may say something about her, it also says something about me. If I'm threatening, perhaps it's because when I see this person, without even being aware of it, my own anxiety is mobilized, and the way I manage my anxiety may be to act tough towards the patient: to deflect the process. Maybe the patient impresses me and I have to deal with that feeling. I therefore accept, methodologically, that I don't know who this anxiety belongs to. The patient is the one who describes it and to be in the here and now means considering that it is a product of the now, of the situation, of our encounter, of the patient's contact with me and of my contact with the patient: this is what produces anxiety. Let's put the anxiety the patient feels in the middle between us and sort it out! What is it for her? What it is for me? What has she understood about herself? What has she understood about me? What have I understood about her? What have I understood about myself? What about me might be worrying her? What about her might be worrying me? In this way, we have at least some small chance of getting ourselves out of our ruts: our beaten paths marked by ideas such as "She's someone who would be anxious as soon as a man approached her or talked to her", while I represent myself as someone who can only be tender, kind and supportive, who could never scare anyone. If this were the case, each of us would have confirmation of our position and the beliefs we have about ourselves – the so-called personality function – and the novelty of the situation would not be taken into account at all. Consequently, the therapist's self-disclosure serves a purpose: it allows us to describe what we are feeling, where necessary, in a brief, discreet way, without letting it become the figure that captures the client's attention and distracts him from his focus on the figure he is constructing. I discreetly use what I may be feeling as one of the materials the client may use to construct the figure being developed. I only conceive of this self-disclosure in relation to what I am feeling in the present moment: to the product of our contact.

Context: Every year, in a relaxed summer atmosphere, Institut Français de Gestalt-thérapie brings together students, professionals and trainers for an intensive seminar on a specific theme. In 2008, the theme was the "now", and the above verbatim report presents my contribution. I've kept its spoken style.

Chapter 6

A Background to "The Field"

When Perls and Goodman refer to "the field" they make it clear that they are referring to the organism/environment field. In doing so, they take for granted what is implied but not adequately spelled out in this expression. What I intend to do here is to unpack it, without attempting to elaborate it or develop it in new directions.

Every field is the "field of . . .". Here, of a given organism and its environment. "*The* field", as such, is merely an operational concept because the field has to be defined in relation to somebody or something. The field always has an organizing principle: the visual field of the eye, the field of consciousness of a mind, the psychological field, a domain organized by the discipline of psychology, the battlefield of a particular war, and so on.

The use of the term "organism" rather than "person" or "subject" implies that this field is defined by the body within it. No environment has meaning except through the body, in the flesh, via continual contact.

The "organism/environment field" is not the same as the "self/world field"; that is, this expression does not imply exclusive reference to the self. Hence it is possible to speak of the field of a particular person or client (organism) and his or her environment. Here we are faced an apparent paradox which is, in fact, merely one aspect of the complexity of the Human Sciences: as Edgar Morin (1986) put it, we are part of but not part of. As he pointed out, in order to be able to see ourselves as part of nature, we have to "withdraw from it" (p. 194). We have to be actor *and* observer. I may be able to conceive of the other as an organism with an environment, but I experience him or her only as environment, part of my own environment. The constructivist approach has to be linked to the objectivist approach in a dialectical to-and-fro tension, rather than merged together in some impossible synthesis.

Using the term "organism/environment field" emphasizes that there is a link between the organism and its environment, expressed by the diagonal slash. The location of this experience between the two poles of the field is called the "contact boundary" since it is the site of the movements of differentiation and integration that animate the field, and simultaneously unify it as a totality and limit it by

DOI: 10.4324/9781003515760-7

delineating its borders. It is these operations that gestalt therapy refers to as "contact", which is a concept fundamental to the Gestalt approach.

1.   Field or Field of . . .

We have Gestalt psychologists such as Köhler, Koffka and Wertheimer to thank for introducing the concept of field into the Human Sciences in general, and psychology in particular. They borrowed it from physics in order to emphasize that percepts (perceptual entities) can only be understood with reference to a larger perceptual field. Each percept is meaningless except in relation to others, and the perceptual field has to be seen as a whole.

It later fell to Lewin (Marrow, 1977), a colleague of theirs at the Institute of Psychology, to expand this concept in the area of social psychology. He defined the field as "a totality of coexisting facts seen as mutually dependant" (Lewin, 1951, p. 206). One of the consequences he drew from this, the source of much debate at the time, was his assertion that behaviour can be defined as a function of both the personality and the environment, and even that the environment is a function of the personality and the personality is a function of the environment. These assertions are almost axiomatic for the modern gestalt therapist.

Lewin describes the field in terms of a number of principles. Malcolm Parlett (1991) has elaborated five of the essential principles that I should like reader to review with some care. I shall therefore only outline some additional considerations here.

For Lewin, the concept of field means a "life space" as lived phenomenologically by a given subject. He sees this life space, with all the ambiguities associated with the idea of space, as an affective space; hence, anything occurring within this life space is immediately perceived as desirable or not. The field is constructed by the *valences* of beings and objects: valence is a force which attracts or repels. But Lewin located valence "inside the head" (Lewin, 1951, p. xx) of the particular subject rather than within the environment as such or in the interaction between organism and environment. Hence it would not be a particular person who was desirable or who had a certain valence, but the desire, sexual for example, of a subject for that person. Here we can see once again the opposition between the "id" conceptualized in Freudian terms as a drive, and Goodman's concept which relocates it as the "id of the situation". This is why I draw on the work of Gibson (1979), who built on Lewin's ideas, in developing the concept of the "id of the situation" (Robine, 2004, p. xx). Gibson refined the concept of valence by adding the notion of *affordance*; that is, the desirability, accessibility, availability, and usability of elements of the environment (Gibson, 1979, pp. 67–82).

For Lewin, the human or animal organism enjoys freedom of movement within its field. Here we see again the ambiguity mentioned above which leads inexorably to the conflation and confusion of two types of space, phenomenological life space and physical space. But, as a number of commentators have pointed out, it is life itself, and not Lewin, which frequently superimposes our experience of space on our experience of the field.

As the field is composed of an organism (in perpetual movement) and an environment (also perceived dynamically), it is animated in a constantly changing process. This change owes as much to the movements imprinted on it by the organism as to variations within the environment and the changing nature of situations. Thus behaviour should be seen similarly not as a direct result of the past but as the outcome of the totality of the current situation (the principle of contemporaneity; i.e. simultaneous occurrence).

The field is made up of everything which is relevant to a subject at a specific time: "What is real is what has consequences", as Lewin wrote (Lewin, 1935, p. 19). But since Lewin was well aware that subjects do not always have knowledge of all possible factors which might be relevant and affect their experience, he was forced to acknowledge that the field (which he believed to be subjective and "in the head" of the particular subject) might involve elements completely outside of the person's psyche. I can illustrate this by taking the example of asbestos whose effects within the "life space" of numerous people were completely unknown and imperceptible for a long time. Nevertheless, asbestos formed part of their field. Some argue that the same holds true of the radio waves and microwaves which constantly pass through us due to the proliferation of emitters and receivers around us. Is a particular subject's field limited to his or her field of awareness or can it be extended to the experiential field, if we posit that, like the Moebius strip which has only one side and one boundary component, there is no separation between conscious and non-conscious experience?

What I have gleaned from this brief survey of Lewin's approach to the field is that the field is always the field of someone or something. But saying that the field is someone's field is not to claim that a person's field means the field of consciousness. Just as a specialist may detect asbestos in the life space of someone who is not aware of it, an "educated arbitrator"[1] may note elements or factors in a given person's field which may affect their behaviour even though they are unaware of them.

I also note that some of Lewin's formulations (field = space, for example) may encourage readers to think of the field as an entity capable of existing independently of the individual. Here my reading of Lewin differs slightly from that suggested by Frank Staemmler in "A Babylonian Confusion" (Staemmler, 2006a), and rather more from that of Gilles Delisle (1998, p. 99) who writes about "introjected micro-fields" and thus transforms the field into a consumable object. The field has to be thought of as an experience. One cannot introject an experience since introjection itself is a form of experience.

Finally, if the field always has to be seen as "the field of" someone, it becomes unthinkable to maintain that one person may have a field in common with someone else. There may be common elements, for example in the visual field or the field of consciousness, but if we accept the definition of the field proposed by Gestalt psychologists cited above (No percept has meaning other than in relation to others, the field of perception should be seen as a whole), or by Lewin or gestalt therapists, these so-called common elements extracted from a unified and unifying whole are not enough to constitute a bi-personal field unless we move from a psychological to a sociological definition of the field.

2.   Organism

The use of the term "organism" may seem slightly disconcerting. However, we should remember that it was dear to Goldstein (Goldstein, 1939; Hall and Lindzey, 1957), who was heavily influenced by Gestalt psychology well before Lewin, and to whom Perls acted as assistant for some time. We might be tempted to replace it by other, more familiar, concepts such as subject, person, agent or individual. However, I can see how Goldstein's use of this concept is linked to his desire to break with a purely mentalist conception of the field (Lewin's *in the head* perhaps) and adopt an embodied position. Lewin, as we have seen, was already speaking of affect. Is it possible to think of affect without the body? He also wrote of the space within which the human or animal moves about. How can we conceive of motor functions without a body? The structuring of the field, also called the construction of the figure/ground relation, always has an element of movement, even if only directing one's gaze or lending one's ear.

We find the same concern in Merleau-Ponty who, through his concept of "flesh" (Merleau-Ponty, 1964, p. 54), stresses the body's relationship with the world, particularly through perception and motor functions, which is what produces meaning.

The body is at the centre of all experience, it is the alpha and the omega, the irreducible dimension and essential component of the field which it forms with the environment. Replacing the concept of body with the broader concept of subject or person restricts the meaning of the expression. Similarly, replacing the concept of "environment" by the narrower one of "the other", even if the other is the most interesting figure in our lived environment, introduces a bias which gets in the way of a true understanding of the principle.

An idea which gestalt therapists have begun to use ever since the concept of the "id of the situation" (Perls, Hefferline and Goodman, 1951, p. 182) saw daylight, and which in my view rests on a misunderstanding, is that the id of the situation is a joint or common id not attributable to either party. It is true that there is a lack of differentiation in the id of the situation, but a lack of differentiation is not at all the same as communality since there is no such thing as a common field. The concept of the "id of the situation" as I understand it – although it marks such a rupture with our cultural paradigms that it is easy to see how misapprehensions arise – sees the origin of meanings, drives, appetites and meanings within the situation here-and-now and not in "the deepest recesses of the human being" where Groddeck and Freud located it with their hypothesis of a "reservoir of drives" (Groddeck, 1923/1979; Freud, 1923/1960). This delocalization goes hand in hand with the principle of contemporaneity discussed above. But these desires, drives and appetites can only exist – etymologically, *ex-sistere*, "be outside" – to the extent that they are felt *within the body* in the form of sensations which will become orientations of meaning.

Another equally common error is to confuse the body, or even emotion, with the id. The body, and more particularly the *desiring body*, is certainly the foundation of all experience in any gestalt construction. But, adopting the expression Freud used when speaking of dreams, the "royal road" to the unconscious, I would say that the body is the "royal road" to the id. The road which leads to Rome is not Rome itself, the road leading to the id is not the id itself, and in any case the id will always escape because it can only ever be found in one of the forms constructed for it, particularly the personality-function of the self, and in contact with the environment.

Although this may seem paradoxical, locating our therapeutic practice within a field perspective makes us pay closer attention to the body, particularly to sensations (proprioceptions), perceptions and motor activities. Here again, taking into account the somatic (bodily) dimensions of experience goes hand in hand with the principle of contemporaneity; that is, seeing bodily experience as both shaped by *and* shaping the situation.

In this respect, we can better understand gestalt therapists' attention to what is felt from moment to moment. Bodily sensation is in fact the starting point for lived experience (even if it originates within the situation) and it takes form within and through contact; that is, emotion, sentiment, thought, image, gesture, action, representation, fantasy, creation and so forth. I should like to adopt Malraux's (1949) term "coherent deformation" which, as taken up by Merleau-Ponty (1964), becomes: "There is signification when we submit the data of the world to a 'coherent deformation'" (p. 54).

If we accept Lewin's hypothesis that the field is a constantly changing process then whatever is felt must be constantly changing too. However, fixations, systems of habits, and the fixed representations the subject may have of him or herself will considerably reduce the possible meanings that can be given to sensation. That is why focusing on what is *felt*, deprived, insofar far as this is possible, of the form and meaning imposed on it by the personality function, reopens the field of what is possible and the possibility of encountering the novelty that transforms.

This transformation is also what Perls and Goodman called the transition from the physiological to the psychological. When certain gestalt therapists describe what they sometimes refer to as the "contact cycle" "– and which I prefer to call the sequence of gestalt construction-destruction – they frequently use the example of hunger, the feeling of hunger which triggers contacting. That is, the operations needed for satisfying this hunger, leading to final contact and resulting in the organism's survival. But this brings us close to the behaviourists' simple description of the reflex arc. What is omitted here is a crucial stage: transformation of *hunger* into *appetite*; that is, the move from physiological ground to psychological figure. The notion of appetite brings in the psychological dimension of the organism and enables it to become a totality once more. Hence we are no longer limited to what

Goodman refers to as "abstractions" such as the body, the psyche or the environment, abstracted from their context and which can only exist in the organism–environment totality from which they have been extracted in order to examine them. The same argument could be advanced in relation to the transition from sight to gaze, as Maldiney (1994a) has shown.

3.   A Self/World Field?

Speaking of the "organism/environment field" is not to speak of a "self/world field" but to recognize that no organism can be separated from its context. Henceforth it is crucial to take into account that each and every patient exists in their own life context, a field composed of the patient and their environment. I cannot of course witness this experience, but during our therapeutic encounter I can observe some of the ways in which this experience takes on structure, and I may eventually make inferences about how it is structured outside this situation, through the patient's accounts and through positing the unified transfer of process.

Our primary interest lies in superimposing the accounts produced by the patient during the session with the immediate experience that emerges in the session. Certainly the patient's account can be seen as content, but like all content it is organized by a *process* that the therapist can implicitly treat as a figure (and treating the *content* as such as background) even if this content will remain the figure as far as the patient is concerned.

The analysis of the processes set in motion in gestalt construction is thus a constant to-and-fro: the analysis of sequences in the here-and-now may throw light on sequences in the there and/or before, just as processes in the past or elsewhere may enable us to understand certain processes co-created by the patient and the therapist during the session. I am tempted here to use the photographic term "depth of field" which refers to the area within which different figures need to be placed in order for the eye to accept it as a clear image. One's history and aspirations, past and future are enfolded within the thickness of the present moment.

And, as we shall see later, while the greater part of the transformational work of therapy definitely takes place within the here-and-now, it still seems to me particularly clumsy when certain therapists try at all costs to ensure that the patient gives voice almost exclusively to what is lived in the present of the relationship with the therapist. This misunderstanding of a so-called therapeutic approach based on a field perspective also suggests that there is a confusion between work focusing on *contact*, which is specific to gestalt therapy and work on the *relationship*, which does not form the backbone of our approach (unless the two concepts are confused!).

4.   Organism/Environment Contact

Of course the diagonal slash which links organism and environment is only in rare cases a material entity. Perls and Goodman suggest the skin as an illustration of such an entity, but in most cases this "place" is not physical: we call it the contact boundary. It is a no-man's-land, and as such, belongs to neither one nor the other, but is part of both at once, the organism and the environment, without either being able to claim proprietal rights. To talk about "my" contact boundary is nonsense because the boundary belongs to nobody. It is possible to talk about "my experience at the contact boundary", but I fear that the expression is superfluous since *all* experience is experience at the contact boundary. Husserl (1913, 1982) taught us that "consciousness" as such does not exist, only the consciousness "of . . .". Being conscious of something means bringing both that something *and* my consciousness into existence. Being conscious of my fingers on the keyboard makes the keyboard exist, and at the same time reveals the existence of my fingers, and, furthermore, of my consciousness.

By the same token, when we use the term "contact",[2] we should systematically add "with" and even "how" we establish this contact. There are many modalities of contact which differ as to what they can create: seeing, hearing, touching, feeling, tasting, remembering, thinking, imagining, writing, speaking, anticipating and dreaming are all modes of contact, as are planning, introjecting, retroflecting and so on. I like to remind myself regularly of the following observation from the general introduction to *Gestalt Therapy*: "The individual who looks at a work of modern art may think he is in contact with the painting whereas in fact he is in contact with the art critic of his favourite newspaper" (Perls, Hefferline and Goodman, 1951/1994, p. xxv). This simple formulation contains several of the essential components of the concept of contact: (i) contact as a concept is quite distinct from that of "relationship", (ii) it emphasizes the need to know *what* is being contacted, and therefore (iii) the modalities will be different. The "contact" with the art critic mentioned here is mediated through thought, or even by a non-conscious reference (hence a non-conscious contact?), whereas "immediate" (unmediated) contact with the painting may be visual and conscious.

Experience might be seen as exclusively intra-psychic or internal, whereas gestalt therapy delocalizes it and places it at the contact boundary. This has important consequences for psychotherapeutic practice. The patient describes her lived experience in terms of guilt, shame, anger, hate, abandonment, rejection, conflict and so on, lived experiences which enable her to characterize her psyche, whereas it is possible to address them directly as contact experiences. The psyche is none other than the sedimented result of previous contacts and the particular form that this sedimentation has given to past contacts. Psychotherapy does not have the direct access to the psyche which might enable it to modify the psyche; it is only the patient who, on the basis of experience lived in contact, is able to assimilate its elements and thereby transform the content and organization of her psyche.

The epistemology of the field which characterizes our approach is of crucial importance since it the human being in context within an environment, unlike most theories of knowledge which focus on the human being in isolation.

5.   The Field of Consciousness and the Organism/ Environment Field

So can we superimpose these two concepts of field on each other? Our clinical experience has shown that a large part of our therapeutic work lies in enlarging our client's field of consciousness so as to encompass material which might be implicit, unformulated, hidden, potential, added or created. Let us imagine that in my particular "organism/ environment field" there is no room for the influence of the astrological position of the planets on my daily life, but that my therapist believes in this, and succeeds in convincing me that they do have an impact on experience. As far as I am concerned, the position of the planets was not originally "in my field" but now it is. As far as my therapist is concerned, it did form part of my field – though I was not aware of it – and in fact exercised a considerable influence on my "life space", as Lewin called it. We could say the same of the electromagnetic waves emitted by mobile phones, radioactivity and other phenomena which are not in my consciousness but which may have an impact on my experience.

In order to dispel this ambiguity, I am tempted to draw on a definition of "phenomenon" which may be derived from the work of Husserl and Heidegger: a phenomenon is something which is often hidden but which can be brought to light through certain operations; more rarely, it is already present (Tatossian, 1979). I would then say that a person's organism/environment field may be partially concealed, partly undeveloped and so on, and that it may be enriched or enlarged by various means. One of these ways is through therapeutic work. And the other is the occasion of such work.

6.   Conclusions for Therapeutic Practice: What Does It Mean to Practice Within a Field Paradigm?

The consequences for therapeutic practice of locating gestalt therapy within a field paradigm are far-reaching and are largely beyond the scope of this article. If the field is not a fixed entity, it is because it exists only in an ever-changing *now*; that is, a *situation*. Gestalt therapy's rootedness in the now – which differs from the "present moment" espoused by Daniel Stern (2003) – means that the practitioner focuses on the situation, on modalities of contacting, on the processes at work, and on the affects mobilized by both parties. This focus also enables us to glimpse the "id of the situation"; that is, the way in which desire emerges within the situation rather than being seen as emanating from some hidden source in the depths of the subject's being.

The gestalt therapist also makes use of fiction (the representations addressed to her by the patient) as a way of understanding the present contacting, and uses the contacting in the here-and-now in order to understand the representations the subject constructs of his own history.

The personality-function of the self provides ontological security by ensuring that one contact is linked to the next in a coherent process which rapidly becomes structure.

Psychotherapy thus provides the opportunity to deconstruct this safety in favour of opening up to the unknown of the now; that is, by taking into account parameters of the now which are "perceived but not known".

Context: The concept of field is probably one of the most polysemic in Human Sciences. Gestalt therapy theorists regularly attempt to clarify its contours, some by drawing on contemporary scientific work, others by referring to the implicit and explicit propositions of its founders. It's the latter approach that I'm focusing on here, in the context of the second issue of Cahiers de Gestalt-thérapie *devoted to this theme, No. 22, published in 2008.*

Notes

1 Translator's note. The original French term is "le tiers-instruit", the title of a book by the philosopher Michel Serre and published in English as *The Troubadour of Knowledge* (Serre, 1997).
2 For more in-depth discussion of the term "contact" in gestalt therapy, the reader is invited to view the DVD in which M.V. Miller, Gary Yontef, Ph. Lichtenberg, M. Spagnuolo-Lobb, P. Philippson, L. Frazao and the author debate this issue (2002, Gestalt-Ed., L'Exprimerie, Bordeaux). See also the special issue on "Contact", *Studies in Gestalt Therapy* Vol. 2, Winter 2007), in which I discuss this theme with Joe Melnick and Mary Lou Scharke in a session chaired by Dan Bloom of the New York Institute for Gestalt Therapy and Ernesto Spinelli, professor of phenomenological psychotherapy in London.

Chapter 7

Towards a Clinical Approach of the Situation

The first theory building of gestalt therapy is more than sixty years old but it is clear that we haven't finished to draw out all the possible developments, to draw all the consequences, theoretical as well as practical and clinical ones. By placing the concept of *contact* as cornerstone of the building they make, the founding fathers change the focal point which was familiar to us: it is not so much the psyche which remains the centre of our attention but what constitutes it little by little, that is to say the contact, the succession of contacts which are ceaselessly developing between each person and her surroundings.

It is no longer the psyche which is taken as organizer of the experience but instead the field; that is, what is unfolding between a given organism and its environment. Although the chosen term "organism" is sometimes criticized these days by some of us who would prefer the term "person" or "subject", it is nevertheless the one I keep for it takes us back to the irreducible dimension of any experience: the body.

And what about the environment? The environment that we talk about here is not an absolute entity but, in the phenomenological perspective that gestalt therapy opted for, it is what makes an environment for oneself. This means that THE field doesn't exist, what exists is an *organism/environment field*, i.e. what is made of a given organism and its environment. "My" field is not "your" field because my experience of the environment is not your experience of the environment, even if we momentarily have a common environment. For instance, I could say that if we are in the same room, let's say even in an environment which may seem common, none of us has the same visual field, none of us has the same affective and relational field, none has the same neighbours . . . and of course our "organisms" are distinct. I therefore state as presupposed that not only there exists no *objectifiable* field but there is not any *common* field either.

Even if Perls and Goodman place the question of the field in the centre of their theoretical apparatus, they evoke it only rarely, and the recorded sessions that Perls left after himself are far from illustrating the way this epistemological choice could have become concrete. It has only been for twenty or twenty-five years that some successors have endeavoured to search for a greater theory–praxis consistence and hence radicalize this sketched direction.

DOI: 10.4324/9781003515760-8

A careful reading of the founding text furthermore allows us to notice that the term "situation" is used about four times more often than the term field. And it is by it that an important lighting can be brought to the field perspective.

The therapeutic device, whatever it is, is above all a certain type of situation. To be conscious of the way a situation has an impact on each of the protagonists is also a way to better understand how we could be impacted by certain situations along our history. To be conscious of the way that we can be creators or co-creators of situations in the here-now is also a way to reinstate or reinforce our abilities for creative adjustment.

The starting point for my interrogation on "the situation", and the surprises that ensued, is to be found in a "little" phrase by Perls and Goodman (PHG, 1951) who evoke the "id of the situation" without developing it so much more! This brief formula has turned in my head for a long time in the manner of a zen koan. Up to us indeed to attempt to solve or to understand this surprising proposition which takes us far from the paths established by Groddeck or Freud, far from the theory of drives and of those inner forces which drive us. The "id OF the situation" and not the "id IN the situation". It means, as I understand it, that the id doesn't arise from any "reservoir of drives" but is generated by the situation. In other words, it is the ephemeral moment that creates intentionality and not the archived history or the residual drives, be they sexual or otherwise. The id of the situation offers itself as a concept articulating the embodiment of the id and the given of the situation.

Although our authors do not mention it, this principle could be enlarged to the other functions of the self: the personality function of the situation, since it is by the situation that the representations of oneself will be met with, appropriately or not; the ego function of the situation since the ego function is only activated when the situation presents the ego with a choice.

This concept of situation is so commonly used that it rarely becomes figure as such in the discourse. It is as a given, implicit ground, rarely presented as figural. However, since a few dozen years back, various researchers, in particular around and following Erving Goffman (from the Chicago School), have placed this concept of situation at the centre of their work. It is unquestionable though that the interest for this approach goes back to the Gestalt psychologists as well as to John Dewey. It is not irrelevant either to remember the importance of Dewey in Goodman's intellectual education. But one would also have to make room for the sociologist Max Weber in the genealogy of this concept.

Dewey, for instance, noticed that the situation has a capacity of *control over the experience*, that it is not just a container. Cultural rules order the way in which individuals should behave by virtue of their presence in a gathering.

Goffman (1964) defined the social situation as "An environment made of mutual possibilities of control, among which an individual will find himself everywhere available to the direct perceptions of all those 'present' and which are similarly accessible to him."

The situation is *object of representation*. The subjects adjust to the situations via the definitions that they give them. This attribution of meaning is therefore a necessary precondition before any act of the adapting will.

To act is therefore to treat a situation. Every individual does not only analyse the situation he finds himself in but he truly constitutes it. He selects and cuts out relevant elements to constitute a situation that is going to form the context of his action. In the field of each individual, he will perceive the possibilities as well as the constraints, implicit as well as explicit. Wittgenstein for instance considered that the perception of meaning is part of the perception of things. In this he is near the phenomenological thesis of "implementness" (Heidegger's concept of "ustensilité"), which makes us comprehend in one same act a chair and its "for sitting".

The situation presents affordances. "To afford" means to have the means to do something, to supply something. The concept of affordance, following Lewin's work on valency, has been particularly developed by Gibson and I often had the occasion to use this concept. The work by Gibson, from 1979, has just been translated and is available in French as of this year and its translators have chosen the term "invites" as translation for affordances. The affordance, or "invite", designates the way the environment can be perceived according to the means at our disposal to intervene in it. A knife is as much an affordance to cut a slice of bread as an affordance to hurt oneself. A cliff is just as much an affordance to contemplate a sunset as one to fall on the rocks below. Affordances can be beneficial or harmful. The active perception of situations is thus controlled by the search for affordances. Critical studies of the use of this concept have shown very clearly that the affordances of objects, of events and of situations depend on the intentional point of view and on the system of standardized and socially organized perspectives. It remains to specify whether the intentional point of view generates the situation or is generated by it.

A contemporary writer, Randall Collins, gives in our context a particularly interesting contribution in his work *Interaction Ritual Chains*. The social structure is for him "a chain of interactional situations, is an ongoing process of stratifying individuals by their emotional energy" (Collins, 2004, p. xiii). Pursuing Erving Goffman's thinking, he considers that to look at things from the individual is the product of religious, political or cultural tendencies that are fairly recent but that this ideology is less productive than the one coming from the dynamics of the situations. The uniqueness, singularity of each individual derives from the way that his paths among interactional chains, the mix of his situations through time differ from those of other people. "In a strong sense," he writes,

> the individual is the interaction ritual chain. The individual is the precipitate of past interactional situations and an ingredient of each new situation. An ingredient, not the determinant, because the situation is an emergent property. A situation is not merely and simply the result of the individual who comes into it, nor even of a combination of individuals (although it is that too). Situations have laws or processes of their own.
>
> (Collins, 2004, p. 5)

For Goffman (quoted by Collins, 2004, p. 23), the ritual situation implies a *situational co-presence* which can become a true encounter when it is a *focused interaction.* To participate in a ritual generates in the individual an emotional energy which possesses a transformational power, particularly by becoming a symbol. One of the elements that Collins adds to Durkheim's and Goffman's elaboration is that what people believe in a given moment fundamentally depends on the type of interaction that is taking place in the situation. It is easy to understand how these propositions can immediately find a resonance in the domain of psychotherapy; when I titled my latest book *Le changement social commence à deux [Social Change Begins with Two]* (Robine, 2012), I was myself following this line of thought without knowing it so well.

I call **situation** the synthetic perception of field elements of all involved protagonists, perception which structures the context of their encounter, gives meaning to it and implicitly defines the modalities of their interaction. It is a space constructed and limited by each of the actors who simultaneously are constructed by it and by the definition that they give to it.

Furthermore, it is important not to lose sight of the fact that reacting to the situation is at the same time acting with one's own memory and one's own affectivity, since they are part of the field (organism/environment) of each participant.

To articulate the concept of field with the one of situation, I would say – maybe provisionally! – that the situation is created by the intersection and the interaction of the fields of each involved protagonist. The immediate and selective perception by each one of the implicit organization of all the actors' fields organizes the situation. From the protagonists' field emerge affordances (Gibson) and valences (Lewin) which compound each other to constitute the situation. As Lewin wrote: "In psychology, we are dealing with situation units" (Lewin, 1952, p. 52).

If Lewin though considered that "The need organizes the field", Malcolm Parlett thinks that this proposition can be reversed and become "The field organizes the need" (Parlett, in Wollants, 2008, p. 18). For in fact, as Lewin also wrote (1926/1999, p. 97, original italics): "The *situation* determines to a large extent the valence which will have an effect and the actions which will be done." And a bit later: "'Such and such need exists' is a proposition equivalent to some extent to 'such and such region of structures has a valence for such and such actions'." That is to say, the situation in its totality is organizing the field as figure/ground process, i.e. the Gestaltung.

In the general introduction to our founding book, Goodman writes:

The therapeutic situation is more than just a statistical event of a doctor plus a patient. [. . .] Neither the full understanding of the organismic functions nor the best knowledge about the environment (society, etc.) covers the total situation. Only the interplay of organism and environment constitutes the psychological situation, not the organism and environment taken separately.

(PHG, pp. xi–xii)

When Perls and Goodman take up the characteristics of the self, they describe it as "engaged with the situation" and note: "We mean that there is no sense of oneself or of other things other than one's experience of the situation" (PHG, 10, 4 – p. 377).

I am made of the situation just as much as I participate with the other in the creation of the situation.

Already, Wertheimer in his study *Productive Thinking* (1945) noted that the capacity to restructure a situation, to look at a situation from another vantage point, constituted essential factors of creativity.

One of the principles proposed by the field perspective is called the principle of contemporaneity. This principle stresses "that it is the constellation of the influences in the *present* field which 'explains' present behaviour. No particular special causal status is accorded to events in the past which, in many systems, are thought of as determinants of what is happening now" (Parlett, 1991, p. 71)

It is probably the most controversial principle, or if not, at least totally ignored. The psychological and psychoanalytical tradition of thought got us so used to considering that our behaviours, symptoms, relations are determined by our history that daring to think that it would *only* be due to the current situation is easily unbearable to us.

Furthermore, any clinician cannot but agree that the current experience undoubtedly contains elements of repetition or reproduction from the past, and that unfinished and fixed situations get activated during therapy just as well as in daily life. In the same way, anticipation, future, intentionality can turn out to be a major organizer of the present moment. Should we see any contradiction in this?

The question can be stated in different terms if we consider that it is not just at any time, in just any circumstances, in just any situation, with just any speaker that stored up material from the past will manifest itself. Every one of us, during personal therapy, will have noticed that certain themes, certain behaviours, certain memories, will never be told about with certain therapists, while they rapidly pop up with some other one.

Gestalt therapy, with its essential centring upon what we call "the process", can offer a hypothesis for understanding. What gets fundamentally stored up is precisely processes, schemas of action and interaction, motoric, emotional, imaginary, language schemas. These patterns are not some content but rather an essentially process-based, procedural memory which, when activated, will be enriched with some content, variable content for it is implicit, variable and contextual interpretation. Besides, the structure of dream can be dealt with using the same working hypothesis.

In a previous article and in another context, I tried to understand what I call here the "structure" of the current experience by using support and example from the language. Here, I will rather use here a metaphor to go further in my hypothesis. We all have seen episodes from American TV series, where one sometimes sees a policeman typing into his computer a photofit or a fingerprint and making dozens of thousands of records roll until a perfect superimposition of the facial structure or fingerprint is obtained with one of the archived ones.

By analogy, I make the hypothesis that in the current situation, with the uttered words, with the form of the relation, with the implicit part of glances, silences, gestures, etc. the "file" of history is invoked and then similar structures "roll", which will get activated in the here-now of the situation.

This hypothesis would thus confirm the "principle of contemporaneity", i.e. that only the situation, in its present moment, gives form to the experience and its formulation, and enriches itself with the thickness of superimposition of some past pattern.

> Freedom is not on the side of the organism, it is to be sought on the side of the situation. Alienation is not on the side of the organism, it is to be sought on the side of the situation. Development is not on the side of the organism, it is to be sought on the side of the situation. For our life is participation in the situation, engagement in the situation.

There is no difference between acting in a situation and the being of acting (Robine, 2004, p. 76).

The question is therefore how the situation can be restructured in such a way that the contact with the environment can turn out more satisfactory.

The answer to that question will be very different from the one proposed by a psychotherapy focusing on the individual's perturbations located in her psyche. The situations in which we are immersed lead us to construct gestalts, i.e. figure/ground relations, this is the reason why we are **gestalt** therapy, not a **psycho**therapy but a therapy of the construction/deconstruction of gestalts.

> What counts is not the infantile (Freud), nor the pedagogical intention (Adler) nor the unconscious made conscious (Jung), but it is the therapeutical experience itself. Certainly the factors we just mentioned play a part, but they are subordinated to the actual moment of experience.
>
> (Rank, 1976, p. 25)

Perls and Goodman already evoked at the time of their writings the gap that therapy was to introduce when they talked about transfer: "The therapeutic meaning of transfer doesn't reside [. . .] in the fact that it is the same old story, but in that it is from now on reworked in a different manner as a present experiment: the analyst is another kind of parent" (PHG, 1951, p, 25).

From the tentative definition I sketched above ("I call *situation* the synthetic perception of field elements by all involved protagonists, perception which structures the context of their encounter, gives meaning to it and implicitly defines the modalities of their interaction"), – with the understanding that with "synthetic perception" I am referring to the implicit synthesis of the involved protagonists – I consider that the psychotherapist has the capacity to put to work the necessary shifts for a redefinition of the situation for therapeutic intents.

To make explicit what I mean by "shift" and "redefinition", I will illustrate with two personal examples, which I purposely pick outside the realm of therapy.

I was taking a walk by myself in the streets of Lower Manhattan when a big guy, almost two-metre tall, comes up to me, grabs me by the collar with his right hand and lifts me off the ground, while showing me a coin in his left hand. The situation is clearly perceived and defined by the two protagonists; the situation is structured and the modalities of our interaction are clear for us both: he is attacking me and I am a designated victim for being robbed or mugged. I quickly choose to look surprised and glad, take hold of the coin he was showing me in his hand and tell him: "Oh! Thank you!" Astonished, he lets me down on the ground and I run away. Of course he easily catches up to me and asks me to give him back his coin. I comply and walk away. I have redefined the situation.

My daughter is then around 5 years old. During a meal, she tells me: "Say, daddy, I have a wart under my foot which hurts a lot. Mommy has tried many tricks but it doesn't work. You who are a therapist, wouldn't you have a solution?" "Of course, I do; it's very simple: I buy your wart!" "What do you mean, you buy it?" "Yes, I buy it from you for one euro." (It was still francs back then though!) "So how do I do it?" "Here is one euro. You have one month to give it to me." Three weeks later: "Daddy, what happens if after one month I still have the wart? I still have it . . ." "No problem! If you want to keep it, you give me back my euro and that's that." One week later, the wart is gone. Here again, redefinition of the situation: I defined as the one who knows because he is a therapist, and she defined as the one who deposits the symptom in supposedly expert hands, the situation gets shifted and becomes a "commercial" transaction which abolishes the implicit and explicit references of our interaction.

Up to each one of us to operate these shifts which can transform the situation.

Starting with the observation that the situation is the matrix of identity, and thereby also the matrix of pathology, and that we are not definitely individualized persons, gestalt therapy methodology offers the possibility to contribute through the therapeutic situation to the process of differentiation and individuation. The situation in its wholeness, invites us, from a hypothesis of uncertainty, of undifferentiation, to redo in each session the path of individuation from the parameters of the now (the bodily and emotional lived experience, the contact and the interaction, the context . . .) instead of resting on our archives.

It is also by having present to mind that the infant and adult development, the psychopathology are also the product of situations following each other, that we can contribute to create therapeutic situations capable of putting movement back in the creative adjustment capacity of our patients, that is to say the capacity to recover a certain freedom since, as Sartre stated, "There is liberty only in situation."

Context: In my concern to make better use of the concept of field, in 2000 I began to rely on that of situation, which offered the possibility of differentiation and clarification. So, when in 2014 the Institut Belge de Gestalt organized a symposium on "La clinique de la situation" and invited me to dialogue on this theme with philosopher and psychoanalyst Miguel Benasayag, it was an opportunity for me to explore it further and move forward in this field/situation complementarity which, in my eyes, can be rich in practical consequences. It had been published in H. Cordier and C. Charlier (eds), Vers une clinique de la situation, L'exprimerie, 2015.

How Situations
Create Pathology

Chapter 8

Gestalt Therapy "AND" Psychopathology

Nine Proposals for Approaching This "AND"

My statement concerns the question of the "AND" that attempts to join two concepts that are sometimes considered hardly compatible: gestalt therapy "AND" psychopathology. This question is not new to our community, but it is not very old either: it was not before the early 1980s – in other words, after some thirty years of existence – that gestalt therapy thoroughly addressed this question, at least for the majority of the approach's followers. Too late! Too late because psychopathology must be an inherent part of the psychotherapeutic discipline, as was the case with psychoanalysis, or else it will be condemned to the status of a peripheral reference used *ad libitum* by the practitioners who are thus free to use it wherever they feel fit, more or less happily and more or less coherently with their psychotherapeutic approach. This is how some of us draw on psychiatric psychopathology, others on psychoanalytic psychopathology (from the most orthodox Freudian type to a more heterodox version) of object relations, without forgetting the Lacanian or Kohutian variants, and still others on the DSM.

Unless . . . unless gestalt therapy cannot be seen as a psychopathology in itself: in this case, the "AND" would no longer be justified. This is what we must examine, without claiming to provide an exhaustive treatment of the issue.

1

Psychopathology, according to the traditional definition, is "the discipline of studying mental illnesses from a psychological point of view, whose results are used for therapeutic ends". This "bad" definition offered by any dictionary is based on the notion of "mental illness", and we all know how questionable this concept is. Despite Canguilhem's authoritative works on "The Normal and the Pathological", the debate is far from closed. This definition effectively situates psychopathology in the medical domain, whereas in my opinion it belongs to a multidisciplinary field including – besides medicine and psychiatric medicine in particular – psychology, philosophy and sociology, to cite only a few major disciplines.

But whatever the approach, it will be tinged with the medical model and its two-stroke engine of diagnosis and treatment. It won't be a question of refuting

DOI: 10.4324/9781003515760-10

the legitimacy of the very principle of diagnosis, and gestalt therapists proceed with their own diagnostic methods, to which I will return later. But it is important to observe and to remember that no diagnostic method exists that is not linked to a choice of possible therapeutic intervention. In other words, in some respects *therapy precedes diagnostic knowledge*, which we call diagnosis, even if the approach appears to proceed in the opposite order. However, many psychopathologies have claimed to be virtually independent disciplines, with a status close to that of "objective sciences", with hardly any concern for the epistemology of situations that allowed the data to be collected.

2

As far as I know, no psychopathology has been able to avoid objectifying the patient, even the most phenomenological, existential or humanist among them. None of them have really considered the relational field constituted with the practitioner, situation, pathos and atmosphere. We are well aware, in reference to field perspective, to what extent the separation between the internal world and the external world comes from an arbitrary theoretical choice, and that the diagnostic attributions made by specialists to the place of their patients often arises from contextual or projected phenomena. Gabriel García Márquez[1] superbly illustrated this in one of his short stories, and David Rosenhan[2] carried out a study that corroborated García Márquez's empirical, dramatized observation.

If our practice is indeed a psychotherapeutic practice, and if, from among these possibilities, we have opted for gestalt therapy (in particular the branch that favours the paradigm of field and situation), we are thus confronted with the problem of finding a psychopathological basis that is consistent with this perspective. The issue is open for discussion, and I would like to mention several possible directions.

3

Kurt Lewin, who went furthest in importing "field theory" from the realm of physics into that of social sciences, also developed an accompanying methodological model, which he called "action research". His approach differs from applied research, which aims to provide actors with points of reference based on a position of knowledge in order to develop their policies, establish evaluations and diagnoses, and make predictions. Lewin advocates non-exteriority in relation to the object: in other words, a break with classical notions of scientific work. The knowledge gained through an action-research perspective is indivisible from the conditions in which it emerged, which provide it with meaning. Practitioners are thus trained in effective social perception, since they belong to the field of phenomena and cannot study these phenomena without interacting with them.

Action research therefore has an ethical dimension: we cannot do whatever we please with or to people in order to acquire knowledge, and ethics cannot be separated from epistemology. The act of acquiring knowledge implies a certain mode of relating to the other (here, a transformational mode), which rules out the will to reduce the other to a mere reflection of ourselves or to subject him or her to our desires; on the contrary, this mode aims for the subject to be independent in our interaction.

Scientific knowledge aims to be objective, neutral and universal, understood as an independent object, indifferent to the ends to which it may serve. There is no relation between epistemological and ethical questions.

Insofar as the type of knowledge does not concern an object separated from the subject but rather its relation with the subject, knowledge is indivisible from the experience through which we gained it. The Lewinian model, in my view, should serve as a reference for us in our approach.

4

For Perls and Goodman, this Lewinian proposal becomes:

> [. . .] from the beginning the patient is an active partner in the work, a trainee in psychotherapy. And the emphasis is shifted from the rather comfortable sentiment that he is sick to the sentiment that he is learning something, for obviously psychotherapy is a humane discipline, a development of Socratic dialectic.[3]

In contemporary gestalt therapy, the dialogical movement placed a particular emphasis on this diagnostic mode. It is especially present in the work of Gary Yontef and Lynne Jacobs in Los Angeles, as well as that of Frank Staemmler in Germany, who devoted the entire second part of his 2004 publication to his work on this theme.[4] This is not the place to debate the differences between the dialogical position and that based on a phenomenological conception of the field; a series of debates have already taken place on this subject with each of these three authors during their teaching stays in France.[5] Nevertheless, we have something to take away from their approach that I would gladly qualify as the median point between the classic intrapsychic reference and a radical field position. Could it perhaps be a required passage to reaching this ideal formulation to come?

5

The choice that we must make is situated between a psychotherapeutic position, which stems from a clinical approach; and a therapeutic position: in other words, a specific mode of encounter with a transformative aim, which could also support psychopathological knowledge. If we choose the first option, psychotherapy is considered a type of applied psychology or psychopathology; in the second case, it is a specific, independent discipline at the crossroads between several disciplines, which allows it to take a dialectical approach to complexity. However – and I insist on this point – I believe that there is a place and perhaps even a need for these two modes, especially since there is sometimes only a fine line dividing them.

Why distinguish between the clinical approach and the psychotherapeutic approach? Let us consider the definition of the clinical approach proposed by Alex Mucchielli:

> The clinical approach consists in considering the subject (an individual, group or institution) within their historical and existential singularity in order to understand them as a whole through a personal relationship built up with this subject. This approach leads the researcher to an in-depth examination of an individual situated case. The approach generally leads to the formulation of a diagnosis of the case under consideration.[6]

In the clinical approach, priority is placed on the subject, within their existential singularity, and this subject is fundamentally the product of their history. This approach is inherently causal, even if the causality is not systematically linear, may depend on multiple factors, and – as systemic epistemology has taught us – may be circular. The patient is a product of their history and therefore appears to us essentially by functioning in an ego mode rooted in the personality function. Even if the present situation calls more for certain facets to be manifested, to the detriment of others, the articulation between the now and the past will usually orient the practitioner toward understanding present phenomena within a transferential register. The present repeats or reproduces, and this repetition opens the way for healing.

Without questioning the value of historicity, if only because patients are happy to hold onto it as a justifying system, I orient my listening differently, and all I attribute to history is a value of learned forms. My attention as a psychotherapist offers this ephemeral ego function in its links with the id function. The id, although it is rarely explicit and requires a significant amount of work to unfold, is always present and at work in every word pronounced, every intonation, every slight movement, every posture displayed. Clothed in the colours of history is certainly one way of reading it, but also and especially clothed (at least according to the theoretical choice I've made) in the colours of the situation here and now. This "id of the situation"[7] that evokes this undifferentiated "you and me and the situation" that we will try to untangle within an unceasing individuation that must be constantly revisited as the situation develops. To use Bachelard's wording, "The spiritual efficiency of two simultaneous consciousnesses, united by the consciousness of their encounter, suddenly escape from the viscous, continuous causality of things. The encounter creates us: we were nothing – or nothing but things – before being united."[8] It is the id of the situation that allows the shift from the objectification of the being to its existence. It is the id's openness and attentiveness that give life. The id is orientation-manipulation toward an unknown "next". But in no time the personality function will show up to clothe the system of representations and imagination (linked just as much to history as to the perception of the now of the situation) with "convenient" forms that are consistent with what is already known. It is there that I consider the most essential part of psychotherapy's therapeutic work to reside, joining the Freudian intuition recalled by Perls and Goodman: "The ego as part of the id" or "The ego that is part of the id is strong; the ego cut off from the id is weak".[9]

The id evokes the "here, now and next", to borrow the terms dear to Goodman. The present moment is at the crossroads between the past that is no longer and the future that is not yet. The traditional clinical attitude willingly emphasizes the past as having produced the now; gestalt therapy prefers to accent the transformational abilities, and therefore emphasizes what is yet to come. Resources should be diagnosed in the now of the situation and, as such, the phenomenological position of setting aside as many preconceived notions concerning the "there" of what there is here, in the present, proves essential and leads to the clarification – in other words, the unfolding – of the instant. And this instant is encounter: I am produced by you and you are produced by me. You affect me and I affect you simultaneously, without any order of priority. My plan is created in your presence just as your plan is created in mine. "If by chance we find each other, it's beautiful. If not [. . .]"[10] . . . If not, it is a sign that we have not put our prejudices far enough aside, and when I say "we", I am thinking first and foremost of the psychotherapist, since we cannot expect this positioning on the part of the patient.

6

In this respect, psychopathology can only be a psychopathology of its actors. It studies representations, emotions, behaviours and processes through the experience of those who become aware of it. If the clinical model claims to understand a human system without trying to change it, and the ethnographer's model recommends observing without aiming to change (since for the ethnographer, the organization must be deciphered and understood without being [too] disturbed), the psychotherapist's model is inseparable from the unceasing transformation of the actors acted upon by the encounter.

To use other terms that I recommended in another context, this involves shifting away from a monadic psychology: that is to say, from a one-person psychology to a two-person psychology. And this psychopathology can only be a psychopathology of movements of the field and of their inflexions – in other words, a psychopathology of contacting; a psychopathology of the presence in the world; a psychopathology of the modes of connection with others and with the world.

7

I would like to quote Dan Bloom, a member of the New York Institute for Gestalt Therapy and former student of Laura Perls, Isadore From and Richard Kitzler, among others:

Gestalt diagnosis is an hypothesis about contact, containing an experiment that enables its own evaluation; diagnosis and therapy are identical. For example: "I notice that when you say the word 'mother,' your voice drops, and I lean forward in my chair. Would you say your sentence again and notice how it sounds to you? What do you experience?" The diagnosis is the "noticing that", which is itself the beginning of the experiment, the therapeutic intervention. As the experiment continues, it informs the developing diagnosis and enables further experiment. Thus, diagnosis becomes experiment, which then becomes further diagnosis, and so on, in a graceful rhythm of contact.[11]

This illustrates Perls and Goodman's surprising assertion that "the diagnosis and the therapy are the same process".[12]

8

Psychology is the study of creative adjustments. Its theme is the ever-renewed transition between novelty and routine, resulting in assimilation and growth. Correspondingly, abnormal psychology is the study of the interruption, inhibition and other accidents in the course of creative adjustment. [. . .] [W]e shall analyze the various neurotic characters as stereotyped patterns limiting the flexible process of creatively addressing the novel.[13]

If gestalt therapy intends to approach psychopathological facts as variations on creative adjustment and the construction of forms in the sense of restricting them, the gestalt therapist is led to work – as Goodman suggests – much more like an art critic or a literary critic[14] than like a doctor.

Along the same lines, following the suggestion Goodman makes in "What is Man?",[15] psychopathology may be approached as a study of the variations and restrictions of curiosity, as Michael V. Miller set out to do.[16] This is also a way to extend the project of gestalt therapy, whose founding work's subtitle is "Excitation and growth in the human personality". Contact with the novel stimulates curiosity, and the various forms of restricting curiosity generate diverse forms of flexing contact. Curiosity as a connecting element is as legitimate as any other underlying theme chosen to construct a psychopathological approach: the libido and its uncertainties could be another such theme, as could anxiety in all its states, etc.

9

One final preoccupation (which does not purport to close the subject): how should we position ourselves regarding the psychopathologies offered by other approaches? If we consider that gestalt therapy IS in itself psychopathology, does this require us to turn our attention away from the other systems of psychopathological approaches?

Here I am of course only referring to psychopathologies, not to nosography and other classificatory systems that are only instruments used by pencil pushers,[17] pharmaceutical laboratories and other healthcare profiteers. I am referring to systems that encourage thought rather than those that discourage thinking and therefore contain a reference to the philosophy of Man. "The psychopathologist is not interested in philosophy because it may provide him with factual knowledge for his scientific discipline but because it opens up the interior space that is home to the possibilities of his knowledge", wrote K. Jaspers.[18]

These different psychopathologies provide us with descriptions of processes and modes of being in the world, seen through prisms specific to each of them. If we are able to wrest ourselves from the grip of their prisms in order to replace them with our own, or to explore the relationship between theirs and ours, we can only gain from the experience, expanding our potential to perceive the specificities of our patients' being in the world and the modes of contact that are established between us. Their considerations on the uncertainties of the connection, modes of expression, changes in affectivity or feelings, body image, the experience of time and so on, can only sharpen the understanding that we develop with the patient during the moments of our encounters. These fundamental themes may be directly linked together with our tools for treatment and the variations of our presence in the situation, and it is in this respect, once again, that psychotherapy and psychopathology can be one and the same discipline.

Context: This chapter is the edited version of a lecture given at the Collégiales 2005 organized by the European Collège of Gestalt Therapy on the theme of psychopathology. The essential question that arose repeatedly concerned the coherence of the various proposals for psychopathology, from the DSM to phenomenology or psychoanalysis, with the specificity of the gestalt therapy approach. Here, I gather together the landmarks introduced by the founders, which can serve as an epistemological foundation for further developments. This text appeared in 2006 in Cahiers de Gestalt-thérapie *no. 19.*

Notes

1 I have included the summary provided by F. Staemmler in his work *Cultiver l'incertitude*, L'exprimerie, Bordeaux, 2004. "Gabriel García Márquez, winner of the Nobel Prize in Literature, describes what happens to a young woman whose car breaks down on a country road in the pouring rain, and who tries to hitchhike to the nearest telephone. After a while, she is picked up by a man driving a van in which a group of passengers are sleeping, covered with blankets. Since the young woman is cold and wet, the woman sitting next to the driver gives her a blanket, too.

After a while, the van stops. She gets out with the other passengers and enters a building. She meets a woman in uniform and tells her that she would like to make a phone call, but is ordered to join the other women in the communal dormitory. Suddenly she realizes that she is in a psychiatric hospital and tries to escape, but in vain. All her explanations, protests and attempts to leave the building are met with force and sedatives, and nothing works. The next morning, she is introduced to the director of the hospital. He treats her in a very friendly, patient way. She tries to convince him that she only came to make a phone call, and asks over and over to be allowed to call her husband to tell him where she is. The doctor talks to her in a paternalistic voice, saying "All in good time", and ends the conversation.

A few weeks later, she manages to send a message to her husband. The price she pays is high: to do so, she has to respond to the sexual advances of one of the night nurses. Her husband's visit to the hospital – a visit which she expects will result in her being allowed to leave – begins with a conversation between her husband and the hospital director. The director explains the woman's mental illness to her husband. He mentions states of excitement, aggressive outbursts and obsessions (especially that of making a phone call); additional treatment as well as the husband's complete cooperation are strictly required in order for the illness to be cured.

After receiving this information, the husband sees his wife. He calms her down, reassures her that she will soon feel better and promises to visit her regularly. At first, she is confused; then she begins to rant and scream like a maniac. The next time her husband visits, she refuses to see him. The doctor calmly tells him, "This is a typical reaction. It will pass."

2 In P. Watzlawick (ed.) (1981) *L'invention de la réalité*, Le Seuil, Paris, 1988, pp. 131–160.
3 PHG, p. 74
4 F. Staemmler, *Cultiver l'incertitude*, L'exprimerie, Bordeaux, 2004.
5 Gary Yontef was invited to the IFGT in the 1990s and Frank Staemmler in the late 1990s; Lynne Jacobs and Frank Staemmler were invited to the Universités d'été de Gestalt-thérapie (gestalt therapy summer university sessions) in Angers, France, in 2000 and 2004, respectively.
6 A. Mucchielli, *Dictionnaire des méthodes qualitatives en sciences humaines*, A. Colin, Paris, 2nd edition, 2004.
7 PHG, p. 251
8 G. Bachelard, in the preface to Martin Buber (1923), *Je et Tu*, Aubier, Paris, 1969, p. 8.
9 PHG, p. 259
10 Allusion to what was called Perls' "Gestalt prayer", often cited in texts from the end of his life, particularly *Gestalt Therapy Verbatim* (1969a).
11 In M. Spagnulo-Lobb and N. Amendt-Lyo, *Creative Licence, the Art of Gestalt Therapy*, Springer, Vienna & New York, 2003, French translation: *Permis de créer*, L'exprimerie, 2005.
12 PHG, p. 301.
13 PHG, p. 54.
14 PHG, p. 320, note 1.
15 In P. Goodman, *Nature Heals*, ed. T. Stoehr, Free Life editions, 1977.
16 Université d'été de Gestalt-thérapie, Angers, 2002, unpublished.
17 I realize that the expression "pencil pusher" is becoming obsolete. Should we perhaps substitute the term "mouse tickler"?
18 K. Jaspers (1913) *Psychopathologie générale*, Tchou-Les Introuvables, Paris, 2000.

Chapter 9

Shame[1]

In our earliest mythology, shame makes its appearance as one of the first human emotions, if not the first: in the Book of Genesis, Adam and Eve discover shame along with their nudity when they taste the fruit of the tree of knowledge. However, shame has long remained little explored or theorized, and only barely distinguished from guilt, which has held pride of place in both religious and psychological traditions, particularly in psychoanalysis.

Certainly shame is present to some extent in some of Freud's writings (1896, 1905, 1929), but I first encountered a consistent attempt to theorize shame when I was working on the concept of contact in the work of Imre Hermann (1943), a Hungarian psychoanalyst who was a pupil of Melanie Klein. Later, in the 1980s, an abundance of writing in English appeared, partly in the context of research on affects and emotions, partly on varying concepts of the self, and also as a result of clinical work on early disturbances of bonding and identity – the narcissistic and borderline disturbances: see particularly Tomkins (1963), Lewis (1971), Wurmser (1981), Nathanson (1987) and others.

Within gestalt therapy, a number of authors began to focus on shame in clinical practice at the beginning of the 1990s, namely Robine (1991), Erskine (1995), Fuhr (1995), Jacobs (1995), Lee & Wheeler (1996) and others. This contributed greatly to advancing the theory and practice of gestalt therapy. In fact for some of these authors an approach to this concept led logically to a radical shift from an individualist paradigm to an intersubjective perspective or even to a field paradigm, and thereby to a reconsideration of the whole tradition of privileging intra-psychic phenomena.

The Phenomenon of Shame

For phenomenology, what is termed a "phenomenon" is seldom limited to what is apparent and experienced as a given. More usually it requires a real effort of explicitation and unfolding for the phenomenon to appear.

1 Originally published in G. Francesetti et al., *Gestalt Therapy in Clinical Practice*, Istituto di Gestalt HCC. (gestaltitaly.com), 2013.

DOI: 10.4324/9781003515760-11

This is certainly so in the case of shame: this is sometimes conscious and felt as an emotion, sometimes confused with guilt or experienced in attenuated forms like modesty, embarrassment or shyness; it may also often be unconscious, unidentified, unformulated but nevertheless essential. It may then only appear after the kind of sustained effort of uncovering that psychotherapy may provide. Hence it is important to make a distinction between shame experienced as an emotion and essential or existential shame, which, like existential anguish, may form a permanent basis and background for a number of conscious experiences.

Shame relates to how we are and how we have been received, accepted and recognized by our meaningful environment. It relates to lived experiences of indignity, weakness, impotence, inadequacy, dependence, fragility and incoherence beneath the gaze of another: the feeling that, "As I am, I am not worthy of belonging to the human community." This formula encapsulates the double nature of this experience: one dimension relates to personal identity and the other to connections and the sense of belonging. Shame is a lack of recognition, and hence a breaking of connection.

The Shame Which Reveals, the Shame Which Hides

The eyelids are lowered, the head is bowed and drawn into the shoulders, the breathing quickens, the body contracts, the face and neck turn red, or, alternatively, there is extreme pallor along with bodily weakness . . . Subjects often resort to metaphors to describe their feelings: wanting to disappear down a hole, wanting the earth to swallow them up. Thus there is an urge to disappear from sight, to become invisible to other people's eyes. People also speak of "losing face", even though the physical manifestations of shame are concentrated on the face. These bodily manifestations demonstrate the ambiguous nature of shame: how are we to make sense of the fact that subjects express the desire to disappear, at least from sight, while the physical signs they produce inevitably attract the eye?

My hypothesis relates to the showing or demonstrating of excitement: blushing may be understood as the physical sign of an excitement that is definitely intense but is interrupted, as when breathing is blocked. The subject perceives that he is showing what he would rather keep hidden: the desiring self. But this self-revelation is also a source of excitement itself because it gives the subject an opportunity to be recognized in his desire, even if this desire is unmentionable.

The shame which finds expression in pallor, sometimes referred to in French as "white shame" as opposed to "red shame", is linked more strongly to the imperative need to disappear from the sight of other people, being more dominated by some experienced deficiency or inadequacy.

Shame is such a painful experience to undergo, especially as it is often intensified by the shame of being ashamed, that any way of avoiding it is preferable, if need be through other affects like anger, scorn, depression or denial.

It is frequently the body which becomes the justification for shame: the slightest physical defect or at least any characteristic seen as such, any deviation from accepted norms can become the support for this affect. Seeing oneself as too fat or too thin, being blond or red-haired, having a limp or a squint are pretexts for shame;

a simple spot on a teenage girl's face can drive her to shut herself in her room until the symptom disappears.

The bodily expression of this suffering enables us to make various assumptions about the process at work. In fact, all experience is primarily an experience lived by the body in the form of sensations, pre-emotional feelings; it is through being received and accepted by the parent or other significant person that the baby learns to *transform* this bodily experience into an affective and relational experience. This is what Perls and Goodman (PHG, 1951) described as the passage from the physiological to the psychological which contact provides. When bodily experience is not received, and even more so if it is despised, mocked, or blamed, it cannot be transformed and will stay at the level of the "body". Thus the subject will be impelled to reduce her means of expression to bodily symptoms (sometimes termed psychosomatic) or to any other method involving excessive investment in the body.

"I cannot be embarrassed at my own body because I exist in it. It is my body as it is for others that embarrasses me" (Sartre, 1939, quoted by Greenberg, 1997). Experience creates the illusion that the body is for oneself, whereas it is actually what Sartre calls "the-body-for-others".

The Gaze of the Other

When the subject experiences shame, she feels alone. She is relegated to a solitude so extreme that she believes that this experience is "her" business, "her" problem, hers, and hers alone. Unlike guilt, when the other is very often present because it is they who have been injured, shame leads to the belief that the other is not involved in this experience. However, it is the gaze of the other which produces the shame, their gaze and their words. Imre Herman (1943), in the lovely passages he devotes to the eyes ("Shining eyes"), wrote of "the fire which blazes in the other's eyes" which reddens the cheeks of the ashamed. Jean-Paul Sartre (1943) emphasizes that it is the gaze of the other which transforms experience:

I have just made a stupid or vulgar gesture: this gesture belongs to me, I do not judge it or blame it, I merely live it, I do it as if for myself. But then I raise my head: someone else was there, and saw me. I am suddenly aware of the vulgarity of my gesture and I am ashamed [. . .] The other is the indispensable mediator between me and myself: I am ashamed of myself as I appear to another.

This gaze of the other may be accompanied by words, reproaches, but it may also be silent and thus leave the way open to all kinds of projections on the part of the person experiencing the shame. Hence ultimately there is no need for the other's gaze to be present in concrete form: it will be internalized and activated without the need for intervention by the self's ego-function.

What the subject *is* – some character trait, expression or aspiration – does not seem acceptable to others, and hence is not acceptable to the subject herself.

Exposed – or potentially exposed – to the gaze of the other, shame triggers off the feeling of a lack of harmony between one's experience of oneself and one's experience of the external world. "Shame assumes that you can be seen and that you are aware that other people can see you: in a word, that you are embarrassed. You are visible but not ready to be visible" wrote Erik H. Erikson (1950) in his theory of psychosocial development. He made shame (as opposed to autonomy) one of the eight stages of human development, a major watershed in reaching equilibrium between antagonistic forces, lack of which may interrupt the process of personal development.

Shame is thus, to use Kaufman's striking phrase, "a break in the bridge between people" (Kaufman, 1989). Shame cuts off and isolates the subject to the point that he begins to forget the very existence of the shame-maker. However, the creation of a feeling of shame, or the reactivation of an existing one, is dependent on the existence of another who puts the subject to shame. An expression often used by parents or teachers who make use of shame as a so-called educational instrument is significant here: "You should be ashamed of yourself!" they tell the child, a usage that is found in many cultures and a variety of languages. In this way, the parent tells the child that he should feel (and the underlying paradox is: if he were good!) while at the same time the adult absolves herself of any responsibility for what the child is feeling, as if she were not involved in the affect she suggests to the child. Or, in a similar register, in response to the child who declares that she does not like a certain food the parent delights in repeating the formula: "You don't say '*I don't like it*', you say '*I'm a silly girl*'!" In both cases, the shame-maker invites the other to feel shame, but then retires from the field of experience, refusing to accept the slightest responsibility for the shame experienced by the child.

The Gaze of the Other Represents the Gaze of the Community

The way I am, the person who is ashamed tells himself, I am not worthy of belonging to the human community. The culture of narcissism encourages us to camouflage and repress our lacks, deficiencies, our feelings of being somehow lacking, in error, at fault and so on. Hence our experience can only be validated if it conforms to the norms and requirements of our social group. The "rest" of our experience, not validated, not received, becomes shameful.

Gordon Wheeler's argument (Lee & Wheeler, 1996) completes this reading: shame is embedded in the individualist paradigm and constitutes one of its major symptoms: individualism sees dependence as childish and considers it inferior. Therefore the individual is forced to repress these feelings as shameful and is unable to feel accepted by the community while he feels beholden to others and thus, *a fortiori*, in a state of dependence.

One of the key studies on shame, by Helen Block Lewis (1971), had already provided an organizing principle for research around what she called "field-dependence or field-independence". Of course her definition of the field is closer to that of Kurt Lewin (the field as "life-space") than that of modern gestalt therapy but she did show that field-dependent subjects proved to be far more prone to shame than guilt during the first therapeutic encounters, whereas field-independent was linked to paranoid conditions (Robine, 1991).

Hence shame is an instrument of social regulation as the feeling of shame makes it possible, to some extent, to make a pact with the person who makes one ashamed. It was probably this possibility of reaching a pact with the enemy that led Perls (1992: 213) to refer to shame and embarrassment (as well as disgust) as the "Quislings of the organism". History relates that Quisling was a Norwegian politician who begged Hitler to occupy Norway, which ultimately led to his proclaiming himself prime minister. His name has become a kind of synonym for "collaborator", in the pejorative sense that the term acquired during the German occupation in the Second World War (Robine, 1991). "Instead of assisting in the healthy functioning of the organism, they obstruct and arrest. [. . .] Quislings identify themselves with the enemy and not with their own people, so shame, embarrassment, self-consciousness, and fear restrict the individual's expressions. Expressions change into repressions . . ." (Perls 1992: 214).

Shame as a Warning System and Regulatory System

Tomkins has shown how shame can be an inhibitor of interest and excitement, joy and pleasure in the same way as disgust can act as an inhibitor and regulator of appetite (a *"modulator affect"*, Tomkins, 1963). He has shown how, right from the earliest stages of infant development, sensory-motor patterns work to reduce or cut off excitement when it becomes so intense as to be uncontainable. We could perhaps say that shame acts to inhibit the prevalence of a self-function in id mode, to the extent that it modifies those affects linked to desires, hopes, needs, wishes, dreams and goals. When I am desiring I am particularly sensitive to the features of my environment and in particular to how it receives and supports me because I am naked and vulnerable. The ultimate nakedness, and hence the ultimate fragility, is when I am exposed as desiring to another.

In a similar way, in my first study of shame (Robine, 1991), I emphasized that shame appeared when there was a break in confluence, and that a new figure could differentiate itself from the ground and emerge in the form of an urge. Here, confluence should be understood in its original meaning (Perls et al., 1951) as an absence of figure/ground differentiation, a state of non-contact and non-awareness. It may also be understood, following Imre Hermann's (1943) theorization of clinging as an accompaniment to "unclinging", a break in attachment such that the baby becomes sensitive to silence, rejection and the absence of signs of recognition. Self-esteem may thereby be badly affected.

The different forms of shame I have outlined here have one important characteristic in common: they are actually felt by the subject. They may therefore be described as affects or emotions. However, there is another form that we may term essential shame or shame at existing, which is often not felt or not identified as such by the subject. The subject describes him or herself as timid, reclusive, introverted, antisocial, neurotic, and so on. Such descriptions are what Perls et Goodman call "rhetorical attitudes", part of the personality function of the self, which enable the subject to avoid confronting shame . . . and the shame of feeling ashamed. Shame may thus preside over a number of avoidance procedures, and underlie the strate-gies which enable the subject to avoid this experience, to avoid having to experi-ence shame at a conscious level.

There are many modalities of avoidance: burying, projecting, unloading the shame onto someone else, using scorn, criticism or sarcasm, inflicting humilia-tion, demanding perfection, being arrogant and condescending, pursuing power and control at all costs, feeling an excessive need to take care of others, to be nice, to please everyone, and so on.

Shame and Guilt

Traditionally, most authors have linked guilt with acting and shame with being. More precisely, shame is related to ourselves, to our own existence, whereas guilt refers to the impact we have on our environment. To put it another way, guilt is an affect linked to acts carried out in our contact with the world, and involves our moral con-science, whereas shame is the result of self-reflexivity (Fuhr et al., 2000). Psychoa-nalysis sees shame as linked to the ego ideal but sees guilt as linked to the superego.

Fuhr and Gremmler-Fuhr (1997, 2000) attempt to nuance this over-simplifying dichotomy; beyond the simple differentiation between doing and being, they put forward the hypothesis that guilt concerns individual and societal values relating to good and evil, with the associated fear of punishment, while shame relates to peo-ple's values concerning what is important for their feelings of worth and belonging.

This distinction once more throws into relief the isolation of the subject who expe-riences shame and the concomitant experience of solitude. All the more so since both civil and religious society offer ways of getting rid of guilt through a scale of punish-ments which supposedly purge the guilt or wash away the sin, through sanctions, fines, imprisonment, penances, mortifications and so on. But society offers no help for dealing with shame. The subject is left face-to-face with herself.

Consequences for the Psychotherapeutic Situation

Extract from the journal of a female patient in a therapy group:

> The therapist speaks to me in a way that invites me to open up, but I still freeze. I feel a stab of shame at having done something, said something badly. I feel other people's eyes boring into me, I am walled up in my shame. I don't want to stay like this, I am angry with him. I clench my teeth, I take short breaths. I turn hard and cold inside, I stretch my body and lift my head up, I stand firm and I say these words to the therapist:

> Me: *"I feel ashamed, you make me experience shame"*.
>   I am amazed at the contrast between the content and the energy of my speech and my rather low voice. Anger and resignation are both at work in this episode, but there is something indefin-able and different there that I can't yet identify.

| The therapist: | *"How do I go about making you ashamed?"* |
| Me: | *"You're asking me to be something other than what I am and I can't, and that makes me feel ashamed!"* |

I am speaking in a brusque and colloquial way, I am looking for a happy medium between closeness and distance, autonomy and dependence, but none of that is very clear to me at the moment.

I can only respond off-the-cuff, I am just aware of his posture: his whole body leaning forwards to hear what I might say, a searching gaze which holds mine in an effort to understand, a firm and warm tone of voice, mind–body alert to the slightest sign I might give.

I think I see two things in his posture, one is drawing me towards understanding the process that makes me react to what he says with shame, but also his own questioning of what he might have said or done to provoke that shame in me. The idea that he might rephrase or change what he says, his kind but demanding attitude towards me that I have already noticed and put to the test in previous sessions, meant that I didn't cut myself off but started on the work that I can carry on in subsequent work sessions and in the longer term will let me engage in more in-depth reorganization and come to terms with my petty feelings of shame.

What I think is paradoxical is that I had to be confronted with shame yet again in order to distance myself from it and begin to free myself from it. Using shame to heal shame! But it's also the human qualities of my therapist and his total commitment to the work which have enabled me to build myself up over the years . . .

Through this work I've been made aware of two aspects of shame: its dark and destructive side, which saps me from within and stifles my day-to-day life, but also its protective side which in some situations has stopped me from getting into extreme courses of action which might have led to my being excluded from my friends and my community.

The therapeutic situation, paradoxically, is not an easy place for those wishing to rid themselves of shame. In fact, as we have seen, since shame is linked to the subject's feeling that he is not as he would want to be, on the one hand, and also, that this experience is lived under the gaze of another, the therapeutic situation seems specifically designed to activate or create shame in the patient. The latter, in effect, comes to see a therapist because he is not satisfied with the way in which he lives, and he displays his ways of being to the gaze of an expert – or so he believes – who is supposed to help guide him towards a more satisfactory way of living.

Furthermore, the individualist paradigm which long dominated therapeutic theory and practice took for granted the patient/therapist dichotomy and tended to attribute all the competence and goodwill to the therapist, and all the resistances, blocks and insufficiencies to the patient. This implicit distribution was certainly not designed to facilitate exposure of the self's most shameful areas.

For these and many other reasons, working on shame in the therapeutic situation is not one of the easiest endeavours. The ways in which psychotherapists are trained (Yontef, 2000) and supervised (Robine, 2007) are equally liable to generate or activate shame in that the student or the practitioner is placed in the position of having the limits of her knowledge and competence observed.

"The most serious obstacle to overcoming the therapeutic impasse, and perhaps the most common contribution on the part of the therapist to the development of an impasse, lies in the therapist's difficulties with regard to his or her own shame" (Jacobs, 2000).

A number of clinicians insist on the need for empathy and a dialogic attitude in the therapist. These are certainly necessary conditions but they are far from being sufficient. They can only provide a foundation on which the complexity of therapeutic work can gradually be built up.

If shame is linked to a lack of recognition of experience, and maybe even more fundamentally of the right to exist, then these lacks will be the principal themes of the therapeutic work. The philosopher Axel Honneth (1992), following Hegel, offers the therapist an array of valuable conceptual tools corresponding to stages in the development of the need for recognition: *self-confidence* which is built on the basis of loving recognition, *self-respect*, based on legal recognition, the right to exist, and finally *self-esteem*, based on the recognition bestowed by social solidarity.

The recognition of the subject's lived experience and the creative nature of his or her ongoing adjustment to circumstances is an indispensable basis for all clinical work on shame. If the psychotherapist gives the patient to understand that he should have acted differently, she is taking on the role of shame-maker.

The original shame-maker(s), insofar as is possible, should be identified, what belongs to them restored, and each of them relocated and understood in the experience of therapist/patient contact and the dynamic transfer.

For some therapists, the dialogic attitude provides the opportunity for them to evoke their own shames with their patients. Although I would not endorse this ethical choice (at least in relation to shames lived outside of the here-and-now of the encounter), I would not turn my back on the experience of solidarity ("being-with" and even more) that the therapeutic relation does and should provide. Uncovering and accepting each other's defences is of crucial importance. Lynne Jacobs (1995, 2000) does not hold back from revealing her own fear of shame and her defences against it to her patients and using them as part of the therapeutic process.

Therapeutic work on shame takes pride of place in supporting the id-function of the self. The world of desires, drives and appetites is often where shame strikes, and uncovering and utilizing the "id of the situation" (Perls et al. 1951) help to restructure and "de-immobilize" unfinished situations, retroflexions and so on. Being able to be received in exposing one's fragilities, disorganization, and vulner-abilities . . . and being able to work on shame-inducing interactions in the present of the situation, including – and particularly – those created jointly with the therapist, prove to be of fundamental interest.

Also, in some cases, we might consider transgenerational and/or psychosocial work, particularly when secrets and loyalties are transmitted and create social shames, for example class shames, or symptoms that recur from generation to generation.

Context: I was probably the first gestalt therapist to write and publish on the theme of shame, since my first text on the subject dates back to 1990. Shame is now a focal point for many clinicians, and every patient, every seminar, every therapeutic group brings to light new ramifications of this theme.

When Francesetti et al. set out to involve a large number of gestalt thera-pists in the writing of Gestalt Therapy in Clinical Practice, *I was happy to make my contribution, especially as approaching psychopathology through the topics experienced by patients has always seemed to me to be more in line with the essential principles of gestalt therapy than any nosographic approach.*

Chapter 10

Shame in Supervision

"The biggest impediment to working through therapeutic impasses – and perhaps the most common therapist contribution to the development of an impasse – is the therapist's difficulty with her own shame." This hypothesis advanced by Lynne Jacobs is usually extended to the situation of supervision. However, it would be unwise to infer that in therapy, as in training or supervision, shame must be avoided at all costs. Our sensitivity to shame, our understanding of the defences it generates, and the deployment and dialogical opening of these experiences can enhance the therapeutic process if they can be specifically resolved in the here and now of the therapeutic relationship.

A narcissistic culture urges us to camouflage and hold back our shortcomings, weaknesses, feelings of insufficiency, mistakes, transgressions, etc. As a result, experience can only be validated if it complies with the norms and requirements of the social group to which we belong. The "rest" of experience, which is not validated and not welcome, turns into shame.

The Socratic method (also known as maieutics[1]) has often been described as one of psychotherapy's ancestral references. What do we mean when we talk about this method of delivering meaning through dialogue? Socrates showed consummate skill in putting his verbal opponent in a difficult position, trapping him in his own contradictions, confronting him with a ruthless logic until the moment of ultimate humiliation: "You thought you knew, but you know nothing! I myself know one thing only: that I know nothing!"

The issue of shame forces us to think about the issue of support, solidarity and connection, and to integrate these components into our presence as psychotherapists, trainers and supervisors.

1. Shame as a Phenomenon

The phenomenological approach has been able to demonstrate that what we call the phenomenon is rarely what appears, which is experienced as a given. Most of the time an extensive task of elucidating and unfolding is needed in order to allow the phenomenon to occur. This is the difference between phenomenology and what might be called phenology: the Greek root of phenomenology denotes

DOI: 10.4324/9781003515760-12

that something "is to be done" before the experience can enter into the field of consciousness and knowledge.

The same is true of shame, which is sometimes conscious and experienced as emotion, sometimes confused with guilt, sometimes felt in attenuated forms such as embarrassment or shyness, and often unconscious, unidentified, unnamed, appearing only at the end of an unfolding process for which psychotherapy may provide an opportunity.

Shame hinges on how we are welcomed, accepted and recognized by our significant environment. It refers to an experience of unworthiness, weakness, helplessness, inadequacy, dependence, fragility and incoherence under the gaze of another person; as I am, I'm not worthy of belonging to the human community. It is therefore a fundamental lack of recognition and the resulting rupture of connection.

Indeed, shame implies the regard of an Other, contrary to what was theorized under the old individualist paradigm in its myth of an isolated, self-sufficient individual. The other may be openly scornful, in which case the pattern of interaction between self and other usually develops in such a way that the other sheds all responsibility and all that remains is the affect and isolation of the ashamed person. The all-too-common "You should be ashamed of yourself!" powerfully demonstrates how the speaker imposes a feeling on the listener, even though the feeling actually concerns the speaker, who then withdraws from the listener's field of consciousness following this insidious infiltration. However, any connection to the other person – even merely being looked at by him or her – can be amply sufficient to generate or awaken shame, especially when the relationship is an invested one, as may be the case of a relationship to one's parents, teachers, trainers, psychotherapists and supervisors and other asymmetrical connections in which one person's development is fuelled by the other person's recognition, among other elements.

Leon Wurmser, who was one of the writers to pioneer this topic, described three main modalities of shame:

– The shame itself: it is the direct experience of shame, experienced as an affect: a specific emotion;
– The anguish of shame: shame is anticipated as an immediate threat and avoidance defences are implemented as a result;
– Shame as potential: it gives rise to the creation of a style that leads to avoiding potential shame (e.g. displaying a defensive grandiosity; hiding or accentuating one's difference).

However, the fundamental issue of shame is rooted in "who I am": what the subject may consider essential to his own identity and, hence, what he can use to reveal his desire. Because he is seen as alive – and therefore as having desires – and because he is experiencing or has experienced the inadequacy of his desire and his inadmissibility, he immobilizes his excitement and turns his experience into shame.

2. Shame in Psychotherapy

This topic has been covered abundantly in publications over the past few years, particularly by gestalt therapists but also by other psychodynamic and interpersonal psychotherapists sensitive to the dynamics of affects and identity-building processes. At the risk of oversimplifying, for our purposes let us focus on the experience of inadequacy. When a patient decides to engage in a psychotherapeutic process, this decision is rooted in feelings of inadequacy, or even the desire to be something other than what he is. The psychotherapeutic situation itself thereby activates this essential shame, and the therapist's presence and regard are themselves iatrogenic factors. The patient is asked to "unveil" his weaknesses and vulnerabilities to someone who will remain willingly (and ethically) discreet, or even hidden, but who will see them nonetheless.

It is therefore essential that the therapist himself has been able to explore his own shame and put it to work, if only to overcome the stigma of shame that securely locks away access to these parts of the experience. One method of defence against shame, which is illusory but common, is indeed to pass it on to someone else and, in this regard, the psychotherapeutic situation is particularly favourable since the patient will be more and more willing to take responsibility for everything wrong with him. The manifestations of individuation and empowerment, criticism and dissatisfaction that the patient may express to the therapist may trigger the latter's defensive reactions (avoidance, denial, holding the other prematurely accountable, projection, etc.). The individualistic way of thinking still has a bright future ahead of it, not least thanks to patients who are moulded by a thousand-year-old intellectual tradition and increasingly immersed in a culture and media favourable to this way of thinking.

3. Under Psychotherapeutic Supervision

In a situation of supervision – which in this respect bears as many similarities to a psychotherapeutic situation as to a training situation – the supervisor is rightly or wrongly invested with a supposed body of knowledge which gives him the hierarchical status of an expert. The supervisee is confronted with the limits of his expertise and competence, or even his orthodoxy. Given his experience and seniority in the profession, the supervisor is set up as a role model and his distinction readily generates or activates shame. The pursuit of excellence, established in principle in many institutions, is not foreign to our sphere and is accompanied by a procession of side effects: emulation and competition, shame and humiliation, repression and suppression, etc.

I have always been challenged, saddened and angered to hear colleagues from all psychotherapeutic approaches talk about their inability to discuss a number of situations in their own supervision in which their practice was on the border of the orthodoxy of their method or beyond, or which had generated feelings, fantasies and countertransferences which, when expressed, would take the form of a confession. Of course, the frequency of these stories about "the others" leads me to infer that the same is probably true of me when I am the supervisor, despite how careful I am regarding this issue.

Certainly, any modality of the psychotherapist's presence – his remarks, from the verbal to the non-verbal aspects of the verbal, gestures and attitudes, connotations, etc. – can be seen as revealing something about him. This may also be approached as a product of the situation: the interaction between the two protagonists, which is therefore generated by two co-creators without any preconceptions allowing either one of them to claim or be assigned ownership of this modality. What cannot be said says something essential about what is happening, and restricting expression to what is "psychotherapeutically correct" is a sign of the principle of an identical practice: the patient must comply with his psychotherapist's theoretical and methodological requirements. If supervision is a form of control – if it proves too "superego-esque" – it will consequently model an equally controlling and adaptation-demanding psychotherapeutic practice.

Supervision may take place in a welcoming, supportive atmosphere, and the quality of the supervisor's presence is a key factor in building the trust and feelings of security needed to unveil spaces of fragility, doubt, shortcomings or failure. Shame seals off those spaces, and the shame of being ashamed adds an extra lock.

4. Orthodoxy

I find the ignorance of a certain number of psychotherapists and psychoanalysts regarding approaches that are not their own to be massive and worrisome. In my view, it denotes a closure to the experience of others when this experience is not filtered by a system of theoretical hypotheses which, by avoiding all confrontation and any dialectic, quickly starts to resemble religious fanaticism. In such a context, daring to think using concepts that have not received the academy's seal of approval, daring to renounce settings that are ritualized but meaningless or irrelevant in a particular case – in short, daring to engage oneself outside the shelters and trenches provided by the Institution means taking the risk of being despised, rejected and excluded from the society of peers.

> Therapist: ". . . Concerning this moment in the session, I thought that this patient might jeopardize a process of projective identification with me . . ."
> Supervisor: "'Projective identification'? What's that? Do you use magic now?"

By saying that, what was the supervisor I heard communicating? That he has some knowledge of the concept, but he denigrates it and rejects its use. The sarcasm he introduces in his speech humiliates and shames the supervisee. He humiliates the psychotherapist for using a concept that does not fall within his own theoretical guidelines. He humiliates by invalidating the approach that advocates such a concept. He humiliates by casting irony on those who are not able to discern between "officially certified" approaches and esoteric quack-doctor approaches.

Aren't there any other possibilities?

If the supervisee feels the need to make use of the concept of projective identification in this context, in doing so he manifests several different things:

- That he reads and works outside the limits of his school's orthodoxy. Should this be supported and encouraged it, or prevented?
- That he tries to think about his practice. Should this be supported and encouraged it, or prevented?
- That he dares to defend statements that he "knows" (probably) go against his supervisor's references. Should this be supported and encouraged it, or prevented?

Nevertheless, it seems appropriate that the supervisor, in his didactic role, be able to guarantee the coherence of the system of thought of the school he represents, whatever it may be. Couldn't he invite the supervisee to unfold and explain his analysis and the conceptualization he has of it, thereby creating a consistent, coherent form with him, to the extent that this is necessary?

The supervisee's experience must be afforded a fundamental consideration, as must the patient's experience, even if doesn't coincide with the psychotherapist's experience, beliefs or theoretical system. If the supervisor hopes to contribute to the professional training of psychotherapists who welcome and respect their patients' experiences, it is crucial that he display the same quality of presence towards the supervisees he oversees. A psychotherapist who has been treated with no regard for his shame by his trainers or supervisors will most likely tend to follow this model in his own practice with his patients, in "good faith".

5. The Supervisor's Knowledge

Situations provided by psychotherapists often require psychopathological, clinical or methodological elucidation. Issues raised in this way sometimes reveal the limitations of the supervisor's knowledge and/or experience. To what extent is the supervisor able to say he doesn't know something? Does he see himself caught in the act of professional incompetence or ineptitude and if so, what sort of defences will he mobilize against shame? Again, the system implemented by the supervisor will serve as a model for the psychotherapist's implicit responses towards his patients when he himself encounters his own limitations.

The opposite extreme is another position the supervisor can easily slip into: knowing in the psychotherapist's place. The supervisor thereby becomes a super-therapist who blithely goes over the therapist's head and thinks, speaks and acts as if he himself were the therapist, forgetting the specificity of the joint creation of the situation (which is irrefutably personal; as Michel de Montaigne said, explaining why he loved his close friend Étienne de La Boétie, "Because it was him; because it was me").

6. Self-Esteem

While self-esteem is often seen as a psychic elaboration, it nevertheless remains a secondary outcome of a contact process and a direct consequence of the esteem that others show towards us. As a result, handling negative feedback is a particularly sensitive issue and the supervisor must be very careful in order to allow the supervisee to listen to and assimilate his comments, as well as those expressed by the group if supervision is practised in groups. The supervisor's comments may even go against the objective being pursued. In the example below, I was attempting to free a therapist from the devaluation into which she had retreated; in doing so, I amplified her shame. (Several months later, the therapist gave me the following extract from her diary.)

... I describe my work session in the following manner:
"I should have done this or that; I wasn't able to . . ." (Here I keep minimizing my status in the group, at the risk of looking bad.)
Supervisor: "I find that for a while you've been expressing things in a negative form; could you try to express them differently?"
It wasn't very hard to spot!
The remark is an opening and yet I remain frozen. I feel shame welling up inside me – shame of having done something wrong, of being "forced" to start over in a form that's supposedly the right form (the constant teacher–student relationship). I feel pinned down by the others' gaze, walled up inside my shame. I don't want to stay in this state; I'm angry with J.-M.R. I clench my jaw, I start breathing rapidly, I go all hard and cold inside, I sit up straight and raise my head up high, I plant my feet firmly on the ground and I address the supervisor as follows:
Me: "I feel ashamed; you make me feel ashamed."
I'm surprised by the contrast between what I'm saying, my intense energy and my rather low tone of voice. Anger and resignation are both at work in this episode, but something indefinable and different is there – present – but I still can't identify it.
Supervisor: "What do I do to make you feel ashamed?"
Me: "You ask me to be something I'm not and I can't do it – it makes me ashamed!"
My way of expressing myself is abrupt and informal; I'm seeking a balance between proximity and distance – between autonomy and dependence – but it isn't very clear to me at the time.
I don't know how to respond at first; I'm just sensitive to his posture: his entire body completely inclined to listen to what might emerge from me; scrutinizing regard that seeks to understand and doesn't let go; firm, warm tone of voice; mind–body awareness on the lookout for the slightest sign that I might give.
I think I sense a dual intent in his posture: to get me to understand the process that leads me to experience his intervention in the form of shame, but also to

ask himself how he, through his way of doing or being, might have provoked such shame in me. This possibility for him to re-examine what might have been a possible error of formulation or content on his part, together with his benevolence and demanding nature towards me, which I was able to pick up on and test in my earlier work under supervision, allow me to not cut myself off, and instead to initiate work that will be extended to further sessions and in the longer term will allow me to extensively reconfigure and come to terms with my little sources of shame.

I often hear J.-M.R. say that what we support in the process that is underway is the construction and formation of the figure; I would add that for me, his human dimension and his total commitment to the work is also what's let me construct myself over the years.

In my opinion, what's ironic here is that I had to be confronted with shame again in order to push it away and start to free myself of it: healing shame with shame!

Through this work, I've become aware of two aspects of shame: its dark, destructive side, which suffocates my daily life by undermining the background, but also its protective aspect, which in certain situations has prevented me from carrying out extreme actions that could have excluded me from my loved ones and my community.

This account clearly shows different ingredients that make up the experience of shame and its therapeutic approach; for example:

– Shame involves a rupture of connection and exclusion from the community.
– The vehicle is just as implicit and non-verbal as it is explicit, if not more. "My friend, you do not know what impertinence a woman like my mother can put into a patronizing look, what humiliation into a word, what contempt into a nod" (Balzac, *The Lily of the Valley*, quoted by Wurmser). What is communicated by the quality of the supervisor's (or psychotherapist's) non-verbal presence, and cannot be interpreted as "a technique" or manipulation on his part, is captured with great intensity.
– Shame is generated or activated in and through the relationship. Something must therefore be opened at both poles of the relational system and as such, the supervisor (in a supervisory situation) and the psychotherapist (in a psychotherapeutic situation) alike must agree to open their part of the situation and consider their role and their own defences in the implementation of the client's, supervisee's or patient's experience.

7. The Psychotherapist's Shame/The Patient's Shame

One of the major difficulties lies in the psychotherapist's misreading, ignorance or outright denial of his own shame in the relationship with a patient, or the supervisor's in the relationship with the colleagues he oversees; shame is one of those affects I like to call "reduplicating affects" which generate "the shame of being ashamed", along the same lines as "the fear of being afraid". The blockage is thus all the more powerful. The psychotherapist who presented the following testimony to her supervision group took the time to write it down between sessions. In order to feel ready taking the plunge, she needed the security of having it in writing.

Claudine says nothing, remaining silent. Contact is difficult for me, even though I'm used to naming and dissecting words, phrases and intonations. She doesn't fit into the category of what I'm used to encountering. She has a different way of doing things: another way of acting; another way of challenging. This approach is based on silence: not an empty silence, not an absent silence, but a questioning silence that comes after me where I don't know what to do: where I have things to learn.

I feel helpless, not knowing what to do, powerless against something I'm here to discover but which eludes me. Shame sets in: it's there, deaf, present in the background. Of course my qualities as a therapist are jeopardized: it's because they're missing and absent that we're at this point in the relationship, or more precisely the absence of a relationship. This repeats itself over and over in my head; my problem becomes "How to get her to say something". If she isn't speaking, it's because I don't know what to do; I'm not up to it. I start feeling trapped, gradually at first but then more and more quickly. I become an executioner: I want her to talk – my very survival depends on it. During our interviews, when she doesn't say anything, I feel responsible for my shame. Fortunately, there's supervision. I begin to understand the mechanism; I start to understand what's happening. I experiment in the reality of the therapeutic relationship that we call transference and countertransference.

I thought I had pretty much dealt with this problem myself, or at least I thought that through the awareness of the process in place, I'd be able to use what I experience as a tool in working with her. That's what I do.

A fleeting illusion! I now understand that I've only begun the slow descent into my own meandering; now that the first step of shame has been covered, the lower layers are next. I immediately think that if I read this text to the group, they'll think I should have dealt with this a long time ago. Shame brings with it the special privilege of having one's head work for two, asking questions and especially answering them. When we're ashamed, in order to avoid letting others present us with these questions and answers, we ask and answer them ourselves long before anyone else has a chance!

New supervision: I raise the issue of illness, and especially my story in relation to illness. The supervisor, Jean-Marie, says (or at least I recall him saying), "What can you do to make room for it so that it doesn't try to go complete itself somewhere else?" This is why I decided to tell the story of my shame: a deep shame that I'd buried away and forgotten, and which is now coming back to me in the form of pain in my solar plexus.

Before I start to write about it, everything runs through my head. If I say that, they won't like me anymore; they'll look at me differently; I'll scare them; I won't be able to be one of them anymore. That's shame: we don't deserve it anymore; we no longer have the qualities or the love of others we had before. Rather than being excluded, we hide, we remain silent, we keep it to ourselves, we swallow our words and we destroy ourselves. This is what I live and what my client is living: not a word about herself, not a single event that could risk making her seem less friendly, but inside her head she can't stop thinking and analysing herself. It goes round and round in her head and in mine. Today I just realized that my shame is deep: it started far back in my personal history, yet it's so close in my daily life.

I was seventeen. I spent three weeks in a psychiatric hospital . . .

[. . .]

This story is meant to show you what shame is and also how, in the end, at every moment, even the oldest memories are present. Because of that, I'm definitely going to guide Claudine differently now because I know what it is; I've lived it. Rather than trying to forget, I'm going to try to use my personal history.

8. Defensiveness

Recognizing one's defensiveness when it affects the patient reopens the possibility of a transformative process. Ultimately, it doesn't matter what is said, even he is hurt by it, as long as he has the security of knowing that we can work on it together. In supervision, the conditions of security and support should be able to help us address the very process of our work together. During supervision sessions, I often realize after one of my interventions that I may have been somewhat scornful. Even before I check with the supervisee to ask whether this may have been the case, I (more or less willingly) reveal the process I employed and the defence system I was led to mobilize. Initiating the discussion provides a break that helps prevent the supervisee from confronting any confusion or uncertainty about his feelings: the affect mobilized by humiliating interventions sometimes takes a long time to identify, and the supervisee may tend to refuse to think that the supervisor could "aim" to hurt him, since he couldn't possibly have such intentions!

It may take a long time before any feedback can be given on potentially shame-generating situations. This discussion may be initiated by the supervisor or the supervisee, who sometimes becomes aware of specific resonances in the aftermath.

Frédéric participates in his supervision group's sessions, expressing himself more or less with ease, but he feels ashamed afterward on a fairly regular basis. He associates it with a family functioning mode: when he was a child, his mother had a very active social life and often had friends and relatives over, with whom she was always very charming. As soon as the door closed behind the last guest, his mother started making extremely poisonous remarks about all her friends in her son's presence. For Frédéric, shame and humiliation were structured as aftermath experiences: for him, it was clear that as soon as he had his back turned, his companions from the supervision group must have been criticizing him and his abilities.

9. Conclusion

Little by little, over time gestalt therapy has been able to separate itself from the dominant individualistic and intrapsychic conception of the human being that prevails in the various currents of psychology in general, and of psychotherapy and psychoanalysis in particular. While many neighbouring approaches (some of which have contributed to the development of the Gestalt model) contain the seeds – and sometimes even more than the seeds – of a theory that does not stop at the isolated individual, few of them have dared to rethink their methodology, theory, practice and theory of practice with the aim of opening up the individual.

Gestalt therapy, drawing on natural evidence of the inseparability of the body and its surroundings, was thus moved to establish a foundational paradigm: the organism/environment field, which resulted in the development of its own concepts (particularly that of *contact*), method and practice in a radical relocation of the subject-object of psychotherapy.

Gestalt therapy's foundational text (published in 1951) is a product of its time, but while it often still retains the imprint of drive theory and other preconceived dichotomies, it opens up many perspectives that its successors attempted to deepen and radicalize or approach from a dialectic perspective in certain later work. Positing contact as "the simplest and first reality" enables the self to be positioned not as a psychic entity, but as a dynamic of the self-world connection in the constant movements of integration–differentiation.

Over the past fifteen years, the research done on the concepts of field and situation, on the I–Thou relationship, on interaction and hermeneutic dialogue, as well as work on dreams within the therapeutic dynamic, and lastly shame and its clinical treatment, in particular, are what have enabled the theoretical evolution and fundamental practice mentioned above to take place.

Context: Since the supervisee most often exposes his or her limitations, failures, doubts and inadequacies, it is very common to feel ashamed. It is also very common for the supervisor to feel shame – whether deliberately or not – when faced with the limits of understanding or competence of his or her colleagues.

This chapter was originally published as "La supervision en psychanalyse et en psychotherapie", in A. Delourme and E. Marc (eds), La supervision en psychanalyse et en psychothérapie, *Dunod, 2007, pp. 107–119, published here with their kind permission.*

Note

1 From the Greek for obstetrics, so named because Socrates aimed to guide people to elucidate their own ideas themselves, much as a midwife helps a mother deliver her baby.

Chapter 11

On the Good Use of *Incoherence*[1]

Even if it is an effect of the theme that I wish to base my reflection on, it seems impossible to me to write any other way than in the first person . . .

In the first person . . . is that so sure? Is there not a bit of you in my thoughts and in the feelings that live in me? *Tous les Tu et tous les Vous* [All those "You"] who have nourished me and shaped me through our encounters, live encounters, paper or screen encounters, brief encounters or encounters that lasted long enough to become bonds. Is it the consciousness of this that made the French poet Arthur Rimbaud write: "Je est un autre" ["I is an Other"]?

But even if it is not time to think about identity and how it is built, it is however from all these others that I have built not only my coherence but also, thank God, my incoherence, my "I" of odds and ends, my *bric-a-brac* of these multiple "You" that have become I. *Bric*, odds, ends, *brac*. Thank God, was I saying? Well, here is already a tinge of incoherence in my expression, as God has nothing to do with this!

When I first came across gestalt therapy at the very beginning of the 1970s, first in printed form, in English, then in French – I think *Rêves et existence en gestalt-thérapie* (the French translation of Frederick Perls's [1969a] *Gestalt Therapy Verbatim*) published in 1971 or 1972, was probably the first book in French – I quickly sensed that with this approach, I would be able to bring together the various lines of work that I had been using for several years: work with creativity and expression, bodily expression in particular, Lewinian group dynamics, psychodrama, the humanistic approach of Carl Rogers, Rollo May, Abraham Maslow, and a few others. Not to mention the extended duration of May 1968 and its social, political, cultural and artistic impact. To this multidirectional bubbling, it seemed to me, gestalt therapy would be able to give a mobile and lively structure, a spine that would allow all the flesh, nerves, bones and various tissues to join, associate, together compose a sum-total that, who knows, might be coherent? A direction of meaning?

Theory Is Like Wood: It Warps

The second or third form of gestalt therapy that I encountered, which at the time preferred to call itself "gestalt" and not "gestalt therapy", was also the first one

DOI: 10.4324/9781003515760-13

that allowed me to experience a long-term programme. This training was held in the French-speaking part of Belgium and was linked to the Gestalt Institute of Cleveland. Erving and Miriam Polster's book *Gestalt Therapy Integrated* provided the theoretical framework, with Joseph Zinker's work *Creative Process in Gestalt Therapy* at times completing the conceptual framework. The most frequent trainers in the programme were Gordon Wheeler, Janine Corbeil and Michel Katzeff.

During a workshop led by one of them, the group is invited to participate to an experiment: each participant writes on a letter-size sheet of paper, in big characters, an adjective describing her[2] and then pins it on her chest before wandering around the room for the group to see. Already at this time, it is as difficult for me to label myself as to label another. After much reluctance, I finally choose a label that seems to me today to be essentially related to the implicit status that the group has put on me: *intellectuel sensuel*. Not knowing how to express this idea in one word, just one, as had been requested, as I considered myself neither a "real" intellectual – my thoughts, my reflections, seem to travel through my senses – nor a "real" sensual – I was still too retroflected to abandon myself to pure sensual contact. So this double concept of sensual-intellectual becomes inseparable, perhaps in the same way that I am unable to respond or even turn towards someone who would call "Jean" or "Marie" insofar as my first name is Jean-Marie. But my choice does not suit the trainer who wishes, as we wander around the room, for each person to find a partner whose characteristic may complement her own and he suspects that my attribute would not allow for this possibility. Sitting face-to-face, we are invited to "teach" our partner how to live and integrate into her experience this dimension that she supposedly do not have, and of which we are the specialized representative. I do not remember who my partner was, nor the subject matter of what we learned from one another, but I remember that this experience was meant to launch our exploration of the theme of polarities.

Next came the presentation of the metaphoric notions of "top-dog" and "underdog", pathetic puppets from a puppet show that would stage the eternal conflict between a domineering Superego and a whining but winning Id, as is usually the case with those who play "Woe is me!" With these concepts, they taught us the dialogue with the empty chair and changing seat with the goal of bringing together the polarities, as is shown in the multiple verbatim transcripts of Fritz Perls's sessions in Esalen (1969a) and as Zinker (1977) details in his first book.

I felt uncomfortable, already at the time, with this way of thinking and acting and, more than forty years later, I still do. I had trouble associating my discovery of the concept of "holism", having read this old edition of the book by Smuts (1927), and even of the concept of *Gestalt* whereby it is the whole that gives meaning to the parts, with the way the therapist was introducing fragmentation into the client's experience. When the patient experiences and describes herself as divided, in a conflict that she calls "interior", of course it seems relevant to me to join her where she is and to help her to rebuild the unity she is looking for. But to have the therapist take the initiative, in his way of thinking and acting, to induce a division of the experience to better reunite it is a step I am not able to take. This approach does not seem coherent to me, in the same way that the comments a therapist could make to his client about a so-called contradiction or incoherence between the sadness or anger she is talking about, and the smile she is simultaneously showing, do not seem coherent. As though to have coherence, it had to be one OR the other; as though she could not at the same time express both anger and embarrassment for showing this anger; as though the experience was made of parts. If the body can be approached in terms of parts, experience cannot, even if for some it can be tempting to adopt the metaphor of parts to theorize the experience: the inner child, the core-self, the internal objects, the topics, the reservoir of impulses, the most profound or the most superficial, the true self hidden deep inside and so on.

Besides, when I see some of my colleagues work with polarities, or when one of my patients shares with me a polarized version of her experience, I am always struck to note (to analyse?) that the polarities in question could not be considered as equivalent forces. For example, it may be a desire pushing in one direction and an introject pushing in the other direction, so that to consider them as polarities is tantamount to perceiving only their behavioural aspect, without really having access to the experience.

My spontaneous choice of the composite characteristic of intellectual–sensual, and perhaps also the choice that was made for me to give me this male–female first name reveal that my allergy to polarities has long been a part of my world map (*weltanschauung*) and that this way of thinking is not coherent with my conception of Man. This has led me to develop my practice in a way that is coherent with who I am and to find in my thinking paths those that allow me to approach *the experience of the other as an already coherent whole*, even if I sometimes find it difficult to understand how this coherence, more inferred than visible, built itself for her. After all, could it not be a similar thought process to the one we implement when we unfold a symptom?

A Marathon of More than 42.195 Years of Gestalt Therapy: Such Resistance![3]

At the time, in the majority of gestalt therapy institutes and written works, projection, introjection, retroflexion, confluence, and a few other modalities, depending on moods, were grouped in the single category of "resistances". "Resistances to what?" I asked my "Polsterized" trainers. The explanation given to me then was that the major concern of the Polsters (1973) was to *integrate* gestalt therapy – *Gestalt Therapy Integrated* is the title of their seminal book – into the psycho-culture of the time, just as psychoanalysis had managed to do a few decades earlier. And as psychoanalysis spoke of *resistance to transference*, we would by analogy, I was told, speak of *resistance to contact*.

This logic seemed to me more than questionable for several reasons: first of all, for psychoanalysis it was much more about resistance to accessing the unconscious than about resistance to transference, all the more because transference itself "must partially be held as a resistance" (Laplanche et Pontalis, 1967, 421). In traditional psychoanalysis, it is more a matter of transference resistance than of resistance transference.

A second objection forces us to recognize that before Polster, Perls himself had qualified these phenomena as resistances, starting with introjection, which he had qualified as "oral resistance" already in his famous lecture presented at the Marienbad Psychoanalysis Congress of 1936, and then picked up and amplified in *Ego, Hunger and Aggression* (1943). This idea of introjection as a resistance was then extended to other modalities (projection, confluence, etc.) The Polsters themselves ended up recognizing that this was a theoretical error, both on their part and on Perls' part (*private conversations*, 1991) but at the time they eliminated the problem by writing an article titled "Psychotherapy without resistance" (1976). But this theoretical "error" would hang on and, to this day, there are still pockets of resistance (!) that keep this terminology.

A third objection to using the concept of resistance in this way is tied to the fact that these phenomena (introjection, retroflection, etc.) were described as being sometimes dysfunctional or pathological and sometimes healthy when consciously chosen. What connotations would a word have, if it can identify either a healthy or a pathological phenomenon, without specifying if it is one or the other? Could we envision using the word "cancer" to designate all forms of cellular growth, whether healthy or pathological? It is very clear to me that "resistance" cannot coherently group together modalities that can be both healthy and pathological.

A multi-year debate opened up at the end of the 1980s in *the Gestalt Journal*, regarding these phenomena, which were then referred to as *"Boundary processes"*. Many gestalt therapy theorists of the time contributed to the debate and attempted to suggest some coherence. None of them succeeded in creating unanimity; even today, and in the microcosm of gestalt therapy, what was for a time named "resistances" has received various names, some aiming to underline the pathological aspect of this or that modality, others approaching them like modalities of contact without presuming their health or lack thereof. On the path leading to building my own theoretical coherence, as I was reading Binswanger's little book *Le rêve et l'existence* (1930), prefaced by Michel Foucault, I came across the concept of *flexion* (in English, often *inflection*) even though I cannot at this point remember whether it was Binswanger or Foucault who introduced it. Perhaps because it includes the same root as some of the phenomena that it might group together (retro*flection*, pro*flection*, de*flection* . . .), this word, which in linguistics refers to the variation of the form of words according to context (as does declension or conjugation) resonated in me as a way of speaking of these modalities. It proposed a variation of the form of this modality according to the context, like a conjugation that would not attribute health to the past perfect tense and pathology to the future perfect tense. I appropriated this concept, which allowed me to escape a pathologizing that did not seem to me coherent with the whole of the theoretical construction, and of course the sphere of influence of my choice remained very restricted in the community.

Would this mean that the concept of resistance cannot be granted a coherent place in the theory of gestalt therapy? Isadore From, in his foundational teachings, likened resistance to a "no"-response in the face of the threat that growth could represent. The interest of introducing this "no"-response lies in the obligation it implies to wonder about the intervention – or lack thereof – of the ego-function of the self in the regulation of this anxiety, which is generated by the possibility of growth. In addition, this concept personally gave me the opportunity for reflection, not only diagnostic or theoretical but also methodological. Indeed, like other concepts that have proven both their relevance in psychology and their appeal for a diagnostic understanding of the patient, it appeared to me that to use this concept to think, in a psychotherapeutic context, might become toxic. How can a useful and relevant concept to analyse and understand become toxic in accompanying development and evolution? I will leave this question open for the moment but let me just mention that this concept, like others in its family, pulls us towards a monadic and intrapsychic view of the experience of the other. So long as we remain in an individualistic approach, it seems to me more methodologically useful, for the benefit of the therapeutic process, to wonder about how I, the therapist, could be resisting, resisting joining the patient right there, where she is, and not over there where I would like her to be. What could be the threat to me of living the contacting in the now as it is and not as it should or might be, according to me? And this could be one step to approach this "resistance" no longer as hers or mine but as a common production, an effect of our coming together, of which it might be fitting – and coherent – progressively to differentiate the constituent elements.

It Is Because the Wood Has Warped That the Structure Loosens Up a Bit

Another incoherence I was immersed in as I progressively appropriated gestalt therapy, regards the reference to field perspective. Like a slogan, the claim that our method was in line with the field theory started by Kurt Lewin (1952) appeared repeatedly in the words of my various trainers. It is true that Kurt Lewin was cited in the foundational work (Perls, Hefferline and Goodman 1951, p. 277), not in reference to field theory but rather to epistemological precautions; and when a few pages further (p. 281) his name is mentioned again, it is not tied to the concept of *field* but this time to that of *situation*, the structure of which he suggests that we analyse. It is, however, certain that the whole of the foundational work can be seen as an invitation to rethink the psychotherapeutic paradigm from a field perspective. But in most of the trainings carried out in most institutes, before the 1980s or even the 1990s, the seminal work *Gestalt Therapy, Excitement and Growth in the Human Personality* is only rarely mentioned, if at all. Fritz Perls' work became known with *Gestalt Therapy Verbatim* and a few demonstration videos of his work at Esalen at the end of the 1960s and there, in spite of the theoretical principles that were put forward, the practical inscription into a field perspective remains uncertain at best, evoking wishful thinking rather than a philosophical and methodological reality. Coming back to the aforementioned work with polarities, the therapist invites the patient to put a "part" of herself in dialog with another "part" of herself. This therapist, just as a stage director would, organizes this "encounter" from "myself" to "myself" ... Where is the organism–environment field? Where is the focus on the contact phenomenon, such an essential concept of both the theory and the method, what comes of the centring on the events and process of contact–boundary? The person is practically approached as a monad and her experience is viewed as predominantly intrapsychic, which may have led some of us to criticize the individualistic approach, not too coherent – it would seem – with the revolutionary principles established at the very origins of gestalt therapy.

This incoherence between the theoretical affirmations and the practical applications led to the great movement that began in the 1980s and especially in the 1990s to effect a paradigm shift and dare to think in terms of field (Robine, 1990a, 1997b, 2004; Wheeler, 1991; Yontef, 1993; Parlett, 1991; etc.). Since then, these authors and many others have been working hard to revisit the whole of the concepts and practices to give them a foundation, or to restore it, in the organism-environment contact. For example, introjection had been essentially theorized and approached as a modality of psychic functioning, in the wake of Ferenczi and Freud; in the process, the fact that there could be no introjection without another that constrains it was forgotten or had receded in the background. This complete reassessment, aiming for a rebuilding of the coherence, seems to me far from complete, which allows a number of inconsistencies to remain alive and well in our community.

The concept of field has thus probably become the area richest with differences of opinion, based on differing understandings of what this polysemic concept can convey. From the ploughman's field to the geographical field, field of application, field of action, battlefield, magnetic field, surgical field, visual field, field of consciousness, depth of field all the way to morphogenic field or Akashic field, all these formulations have ended up producing a sort of generic term to identify a *virtual range*. They have all contributed rich and significant clarifications, sometimes mutually incompatible ... even as we are searching for coherence. Because the word "field" cannot be alone. Just like Husserl (1929) had shown that "consciousness" is meaningless if we forget that there is only "consciousness *of something*", all the different fields above are fields *of something* or *someone*. The magnetic field is the field of a magnet, of what this magnet attracts towards it, and what repels away from it; a visual field implies an eye and something to see, a field of consciousness requires consciousness ... and something that penetrates it. However, Perls and Goodman (PHG, 1951), as they invite us to think in terms of field, never use a generic notion of field: they always speak of the *organism–environment* field. And it is important to remember that this virtual range or *lived space*, as phenomenologists refer to it, refers to *an experience* that is currently being lived and not some concrete and material tangible reality. What creates environment for me, as an experience, is not the same as what creates environment for you, even if we are in the same space, the same room, the same situation. At the very least, we will not have the same visual field, the same field of consciousness or the same feelings. It seems illegitimate for me to speak or even think of a common field, when a patient and I share, however, intense an encounter, as your experience will never be my experience nor my experience yours, even if I am capable of great empathy.

The idea of "common field" is spreading widely today, also in psychoanalysis (in particular post-Bionian psychoanalysis). After all why not, if we keep in mind that the concept is used with a completely different definition from the one given by Perls and Goodman for the context of gestalt therapy. But what deeply concerns me is that the use of this terminology may create an implicit certainty – even if illusory – of the existence of a common experience, even of its possibility. Is this a trace of the eternal myth of *We* (Miller, 2000)? Of nostalgia for the forever lost Garden of Eden? Of a need for confluence, for negation of borders and differences?

This new theoretical incoherence (or more accurately: this approach of the concept that I see as incoherent) has led me to focus more acutely on the way our founders had handled this concept and to find out in the process that they had also used another concept *at the same time*, which had gone unnoticed, that of "situation". Because what is created with another, or many others, is a succession of situations, in other words of times and places in which your field, your fields, and my field will partially combine, together mutually orient themselves and implicitly structure themselves to build meaning and define the place and function of each of us, define the modalities of our interactions (see Robine, 2015). By definition, a situation is common – a conference, a therapy session, a religious ceremony, a market, a family event . . . – even if each person has a specific experience in the common situation as each experience will be differentiated and hence allows continuous individuation.

Towards the end of his life, Perls (2019) wrote: "The term 'situation' thus assumes preferential status in our approach. To let the 'situation' control one's action is the essence of wisdom" (p. 27).

"Scientific truth has as its sign coherence and efficacy. Poetic truth has as its sign beauty" (Aimé Césaire)

Gestalt therapy is certainly not the only approach in which theoretical inconsistencies can be found. The history of psychoanalysis, for example, is littered with accusations of theoretical inconsistencies or lack of coherence between theory and practice. Among the ones I encountered in my readings, beyond those pointed out by the dissidents (Reich, Rank, Jung, Adler, Hartman, Perls, etc.) the traditional one that particularly interested me was recalled by Bernard Brusset

(1988). To justify the appearance of the so-called "object-relation" psychoanalyses, he reminded us of the paradox present in having forever more elaborate *intrapsychic* theory and metapsychology while executing them through a *relational* practice, as the analysis of the transference is the essential work tool. I would even add that I have always been astounded to see how violently traditional psychoanalysis, particular French psychoanalysis, attacked the main branches of American psychoanalysis (Ego psychology, self-psychology, intersubjective psychoanalysis, etc.), which were accused of being non-orthodox and were hence rejected by the fundamentalists. This form of incoherence meets another: the essential criticism formulated in 1973 by Robert Castel in *Le psychanalysme*. From a sociological analysis of Marxist inspiration, he condemns the fact that psychoanalysis refuses to apply to itself the analysis tool used in its practice, which generates a massive blind spot, for example concerning power relations and the place of money.

Admittedly, critical analyses of a system by denouncing some of its inconsistencies can feed the rigidification of the defences of said system, especially if this denouncing comes from the outside. But they can also be a powerful stimulant to move forward on the path to coherence, which can only be a quest and not an absolute. I deeply believe that a system that would have reached generalized coherence would immediately be a dead system and would also be fatal for whatever would come near it. Nothing can move anymore. When the Rubik's cube is solved, when all the faces have become monochromic as desired, after minutes or hours of trial and error, the process is immobilized, dead: there is nothing else to do but to deconstruct and start again.

About twenty years ago, I led a workshop multiple times entitled "Ce que je crois et ce que je crois que je crois" [*What I Believe and What I Believe that I Believe*]. In this experimental and experiential workshops, the participants were invited to share their essential convictions regarding psychotherapy, their fundamental principles as they can name them (I called this *What I Believe that I Believe*) to confront them to a concretization that other participants could observe in a session and that, perhaps, would be the "true" enactment of the *What I Believe* of the therapist in situation. Do we do what we say we do? Do we behave in a manner coherent with our principles or do we lull ourselves with sweet illusions?

For example, one therapist might say of himself that when a patient tries to put a symptom to work, he is primarily drawn to becoming aware of the creative adaptation function in the context of this patient's daily life. But as the patient starts to talk about her symptom, the *first* questions that the therapist asks are about the anamnesis, the origin of this symptom . . . when it isn't the trans-generational dimension, updated by a genogram! Another therapist might put forward his conception of repetition (of a scheme, of a symptom, of an impasse . . .) as insistence, insistence to manifest pain, insistence to express something that probably someone has trouble getting to be heard, and in the reality of the session, we may see a discrete form of irritation towards this new repetition, sometimes even reproachful interventions. Can someone who expresses their pain be reproached? Examples of our inconsistencies, contradictions, or paradoxes could fill a whole book! I return to some earlier thoughts (Robine 2015):

> What we call the self's personality function is the system of representations that I construct over time through my actions, my contacts and my experience of the world. This personality function is therefore made up of beliefs forged over time; it structures the rhetoric of *what I believe*. What I believe is a construction, although it is certainly based on experience, but it's also a fiction: a representation that suits me and contributes to the image I have of myself, sometimes idealizing it and sometimes devaluing it. That's why – and in this respect it is faithful to Goodman's conviction that the soul (or self) is where the action is – there may be a difference between "what I believe I believe", through my system of representations and verbalization, and "what I believe", which also reveals itself through action, in the unformulated or the implicit, immersed in situations, and which may reveal major differences.
>
> This gap – which I recognize in myself and I notice in each of us, and which I refer to here as the difference between "what I believe" and "what I believe I believe" – is important to become aware of. The consistency that we all try to construct between the different levels of our experience involves continually narrowing this gap. It is also one our supervisors' responsibilities to remind us of this distance, from their outsider perspective, and help us bring it into the realm of awareness.
>
> (Robine, 2015, pp. 227–228)

It is said that Paul Goodman insisted a lot on this form of coherence, consisting of becoming able to *say what we do*, even though we, trainers and teachers, might be more inclined to expect from the other that *they do what we say* . . .

Creation, Progress Versus – or Along with – Decomposition, Crisis?

A quick glance at the macroscopic level of coherence and incoherence might contribute to highlighting, by amplification, some characteristics of a phenomenon. Perls, in his day, was able to leverage this modality for the purpose of raising awareness: he would readily suggests that his patients amplify, exaggerate, a trait, a gesture, a breath, a posture, a sound . . . and the paroxysmal product of this experimentation would shed light on more or less latent dimensions of their being-in-the-world.

At the time that I am writing this, the whole world is grappling with the Covid-19 pandemic. The amplitude of this phenomenon gives it an abundantly macroscopic dimension. "Unprecedented" is the recurring adjective that the media attribute to successive news and stories. Yet the situation allowed Trump to amplify the characteristics of Trump, Bolsonaro to do even more Bolsonaro, the perverts and crooks to set-up their scams at record-breaking pace, the proponents of solidarity to invent unsuspected forms of attention to others, and so on. In a way, it is the microscopic level: we adapt to the crisis by doing a bit more – or a lot more – of the same thing.

But another dimension of this event is that it is blowing up the coherence from which the dominant system, liberal and capitalistic, drew its satisfaction and pride. To make maximum profit, it has its essentials produced where labour is dirt-cheap. The daily, thankless tasks like those of the supermarket cashiers, caregivers, garbage men or the cleaning services are underpaid because they are not as important as the shareholders who are considered the "true" actors of its economy. The owner of billions in shares and securities is not subjected to the wealth tax, whereas the owner of a family farm, which allows survival from a paltry agricultural revenue, if on a popular holiday location, though it has been in the family for generations, this owner is subjected to the wealth tax. The caregivers and the emergency services have, for years, been screaming their despair as they watch their means decrease alarmingly to rationalize budgetary choices for the benefit of other so-called priority activities. And a grain of sand, no, a virus, a thousand times smaller than a grain of sand, is overthrowing the system: all the workers of the bottom of the ladder are honoured, applauded, their importance is unveiled, they are promised (yes indeed) a statutory recognition with hard cash. It had somehow been forgotten that the system could only function if the health of all, or at least of a majority, was assured, only if basic services were performed: garbage collection, daily emergency repairs, cleaning, mail. The building of cars and planes is put on hold to produce medical coats, LVMH or Dior stop producing fabric squares for $200 per square foot and instead produce masks for 1 to 2 dollars, the cognac and whisky distilleries transform their chain of production to instead produce hydro-alcoholic gel . . .

A coherence so well-honed that it produces exponential differences, for example in revenues, for example in access to culture, in care or simply in access to water – for an example regarding ecological concerns; this coherence reveals its incoherence.

And here again, just as I was trying to show when illustrating the microscopic level of theory and practice of gestalt therapy, the emergence of incoherence is an opportunity. It is an opportunity because it paves the way to the crisis. The French Bailly dictionary for ancient Greek, reveals the polysemous nature of the word "crisis": 1/ action of or capacity to distinguish, 2/ action of choosing, 3/ action of separating, 4/ action of deciding.

That's quite something: distinguish, choose, separate, decide . . .

And of course, in one critical and dramatic moment!

When it seems to me incoherent to *choose* a theory that would cause me to *separate* my patient into polarities to help her to build her unity, I *decide* to *think* and *act* differently.

When a society discovers the incoherence of its economic power, when it depends on the disequilibrium generated by a virus only a few microns in size and on solutions that exist only at the other end of the planet, what will it *separate* from, what will it *choose, decide*?

If I draw on the models of change put forth by the School of Palo Alto (Watzlawick, 1975), we have two paths to choose from, which the authors name Type 1 change and Type 2 change.

Type 1 change consists of doing more of the same and, in this case, the problem is often the solution that was found. To make more money, let's have the masks made in China; the solution has become a problem. The individual creates her pathology by fragmenting herself, let's think in terms of polarities or in terms of internal, conflicting impulses: my way of thinking has become the problem. Let's take an example in a couple crisis (simplified at the risk of caricature): he is suffocating somewhat in the controlling relational patterns of his couple and he embarks on an extramarital affair. After a while, she finds out. Crisis. Loss of trust. Divorce within sight even though neither one really wishes for it. Negotiations, getting closer, compromise: he leaves his lover and his wife becomes even more suspicious and controlling. The solution reproduces and amplifies the situation that had led to the problem: more of the same. In France, the original cluster of the virus is identified: it spread from an evangelical prayer gathering. Solution: let's pray to our God that he saves us from this epidemic.

Type 2 change is the change of paradigm, the art of finding a new definition, a new frame of reference, and new fundamentals. If it is no longer profit that organizes our social system, what could it be? If academic expertise of the psychotherapist is not a guarantee of his expertise, what could be? If what happens between you and I could be considered not only as reproduction of childhood patterns, how might we consider it? If I approached my client in her coherent form, hers, which is not mine, what could be the consequences of this?

How Can We Live Without the Unknown Before Us?
As a Poet Would Say

Thankfully, I do sometimes become conscious of some of my inconsistencies. So I mobilize everything I can to reach a new coherence. Shortly thereafter, it cracks and shows some inconsistencies. So I mobilize everything I can to reach a new coherence. Shortly thereafter, it cracks and shows some inconsistencies. So I mobilize everything I can to reach a new coherence. Shortly thereafter, it cracks and shows some inconsistencies. So I mobilize everything I can to . . .

Context: I've always been in search of greater coherence – between my theorizing and my practice, between my professional style and my ethics, for example. Could this be a never-ending process?

This text appeared in French in 2020 in Cahiers de Gestalt-thérapie, *no. 43, then in 2021 in its English translation in* Gestalt Review, *Vol. 25, No. 2.*

Notes

1 Note about translation: The French word *incohérence* sometimes translates as "inco-herence", but most often "inconsistencies" will be more fitting in the chapter. Some of the elegance of the original language is at times lost in translation to remain true to the intended meaning.
2 To avoid cumbersome he/she, his/her and the like, I have made the arbitrary choice to have participants and clients be *feminine* and therapists and trainers be *masculine*.
3 42.195 is the length of a marathon in kilometres as well as – more or less – how long the author has been practising gestalt therapy in years.

How Situations
Create Forms

Chapter 12

Gestalt Therapy as Aesthetics

The post-war Spanish poet Blas de Otero always insisted on being considered as a person and not just an "ill-formed scribble". These words are equally applicable to the psychotherapist's attitude to the patient: "It's important to me that you are a person and not just an ill-formed scribble."

At the heart of gestalt therapy there lies an implicit and perhaps surprising proposal: that as well as evaluating health according to medical and scientific criteria we should also judge it on aesthetic criteria. Aesthetic criteria can be added to those others, or even replace them – why not? We can then see health as the capacity to create forms that are relevant to situations, and pathology as the loss of this potentiality and a resort to rigid, inadequate or outmoded forms, a kind of scribbling.

Hence the founders of gestalt therapy drew their own conclusions from the intuitions of psychoanalysts like Groddeck or Otto Rank: if "the neurotic is a failed artist" then the healthy person is one who is able to create their own existence in the same way as a work of art.

The basic criterion of health then becomes the capacity to create, the ability to create forms or gestalts, and thus define psychotherapy as form-formation therapy, in other words, gestalt therapy. The psychotherapist's ethics then become aesthetics, and clinical intervention into the psyche becomes a clinical intervention into the *Gestaltung*, the process of form-formation.

Certainly, if we look at history, including the personal histories of Frederick and Laura Perls and Paul Goodman, we can already find links between these two worlds. Fritz Perls as a young man in Germany took classes with Max Reinhardt and performed in the plays he produced. He was a keen participant in Bauhaus circles. It was Laura, who spent her youth immersed in German expressionism, who brought the concept of Gestalt to her marriage with Frederick; she danced in the way popularized by Dalcroze, one of the pioneers of rhythmic physical education, and as well as quoting her favourite poets, she would often play the piano, even during sessions, as another way of expressing what was implicit. Paul Goodman was a writer, poet, essayist, and playwright. But all this is background: it does not of itself explain why their theoretical and practical work attaches such importance to aesthetics. I would like to discuss certain aspects of this here, although I realize that they all deserve a fuller treatment.

DOI: 10.4324/9781003515760-15

It was Laura Perls of course who first made an explicit link between aesthetics and gestalt therapy by asserting that: "The fundamental concepts of Gestalt psychotherapy are philosophical and aesthetic rather than technical" (1989, p. 133). It was probably Baumgarten's original definition rather than contemporary references to "beauty" that enabled Laura to adopt this concept. Baumgarten, an eighteenth-century German philosopher, created the term "aesthetic", from the Greek *aisthétikos*, to refer to the science of sensory knowledge, which he contrasted with the knowledge of conceptual objects. In aesthetics, it is the senses and sensory objects that enable us to recreate both meaning and existence, and create new forms of subjectivation. Baumgarten also gave us what is probably still today one of the finest definitions of aesthetics: "The art of thinking beautifully" (cited in Jimenez, 2004, p. 13).

Jean Paul, the nineteenth-century German Romantic philosopher, defined aesthetics as "a theory of foretaste" and this definition is worth pausing over, as it is linked to the forecontact to which we attach so much importance, or the "pre" that Francis Ponge hymned in *La fabrique du pré* (The Construction of the Pre).[1] But even though aesthetic philosophy is not to be confused with the philosophy of art, the reference to art is of course not entirely foreign to the aesthetic approach: art is one of the activities in which aesthetics can be brought into play. Art is not only a privileged form of aesthetics but almost the paradigmatic form. But a number of other human activities can be seen as having an aesthetic dimension: politics and business, religion and advertising, gardening, cooking . . .

Hence today the term "aesthetic" has two different meanings: one relates to art, the other relates to sensoriality, or receptiveness to sensation.

Laura Perls makes the link between them as follows:

> The main concern of the artist is certainly not the "exercise of aesthetic transformation" of truth into beauty but the organization of a multitude of various disparate, incompatible experiences which threaten the individual or society with disintegration therefore are experienced as ugly – into a meaningful, integrated whole, a unity within which they make sense and which therefore is or may be experienced as beautiful.
>
> (1989, p. 63)

Could we not see this as a definition of what the psychotherapist is aiming at?

Kant wanted to reconcile what is felt and what is thought. There are no criteria for judging an artwork because the work *is* its own criterion. For Kant the work of art is nomothetic, that is, it sets up its own laws. In fact art has one characteristic which sets it apart from other human activities and institutions: while other human activities are judged according to their relative efficacy and usefulness in terms of the values they embody, the work of art refuses to accept any such reference to its usefulness or to external criteria or to accepted values.

Paul Goodman, one of the co-founders of gestalt therapy, positioned psychotherapy within this Kantian perspective to an extent when he wrote "the fact that the Gestalt has specific observable psychological properties is of capital importance in psychotherapy for it gives *an autonomous criterion of the depth and reality of the experience*" (Perls, Hefferline and Goodman, 1951/1994, p. 54).

The aesthetic aspect of gestalt therapy locates the origin of experience in the senses: feelings, sensations, perceptions. As Dan Bloom wrote,

> If we understand the figure/background process as essentially one that is sensed, felt, perceived, we can then notice the fluidity or fixity of this through its aesthetic qualities. Experience may then be appreciated for its intrinsic form rather than by comparison extrinsic content-based standard.
>
> (Bloom, 2005)

1.   An Aesthetics of Contact

Contact, which Perls and Goodman define as "the first and simplest reality" (Perls, Hefferline and Goodman, 1951/1994, p. 49), has observable properties which we grasp through our senses.

The authors draw on aesthetic terminology when they describe the figure: clarity, brilliance, liveliness, meaningfulness, sharpness, intensity, unity, uniqueness, harmony, grace, fluidity, vitality, rhythm, symmetry, to mention just a few.

These are terms drawn from the same semantic field which describes physical activity, consciousness, breathing, vocalizing and so on. These terms are not based on clinical, social or cultural criteria but on direct sensory experience.

It is not necessary to have theories of "normal behaviour" or "adjustment to reality" except in order to explore. When the figure is dull, confused, graceless, lacking in energy (a "weak *Gestalt*") we may be sure that there is a lack of contact, something in the environment is blocked out, some vital organic need is not being expressed. The person is not "all there"; that is, his whole field cannot lend its urgency and resources to the completion of the figure (Perls, Hefferline and Goodman, 1951/1994, p. 54).

In the words of Isadore From, a member of the group which founded gestalt therapy, the aim of psychotherapy is to help clients transform their prose into poetry, their walking into dance. As Michael V. Miller explained:

> The accent here is on the fact that the talking and the walking, and, therefore, the poetry and the dancing, come from the client. If it is merely a case of the therapist transmitting ideas about what makes good dance or poetry, then therapy is nothing more than another forced introjection, another neurotic loss of contact. Our clients (and ourselves) already possess an ample supply these taken in from parents, teachers, priests and other authorities. From's remark brings out unmistakeably the aesthetic emphasis in Gestalt therapy and in addition makes it clear that the client, and not the therapist, is the artist who really matters.
>
> (Miller, 2002, p. 202)

Since clinical practice does not rely on any criteria external to the actual thera-peutic situation it is the therapeutic encounter itself, and its own form-formation, which generates its own aesthetic criteria of what constitutes a *good* form. Since gestalt therapy is based on this surprising conception of what psychotherapy is about, it is not surprising that gestalt therapists often draw out their clients' crea-tive potential, and frequently suggest practical ways of working with expressive media – and reject the kind of normative practice advocated by those who see themselves as the official upholders of a single truth.

Our task is to develop an aesthetics in progress as a felt and perceived organiza-tion of experience. Just as artists manipulate their chosen artistic medium to create a work of art, in the course of everyday contact we all manipulate and restructure the organism-environment into meaningful whole experiences (Perls, Hefferline and Goodman, 1951; Dewey, 1933).

Like modern artists, psychotherapists need to "invent the series of positions and gestures which will allow them to produce something" (Bourriaud, 2001, p. 11).

It may be valuable for us to keep going back to the practice of artists who were working at the time when the practice of psychotherapy first emerged: they may have much to contribute to our understanding of our own attitudes and modalities of making contact.

I am thinking here of Picasso who produced his own solution to Husserl's famous paradox of the cube: we can only ever see three of its sides at one time.

In his portraits he restructured faces so as to show all their profiles at once.

I am thinking of Magritte whose famous statement "this is not a pipe" demon-strated, as did Korzybski, the father of general semantics, that "the word is not the thing" and "the map is not the territory".

I am thinking of Andy Warhol who imbued the most ordinary everyday objects like Campbell soup tins with wonder . . .

I am thinking of LaMonte Young, Terry Riley, Steve Reich or Philip Glass, creators of what is known as repetitive or minimalist music, who bring to the fore what is background in traditional musical composition and turn it into figure.

I am thinking of Pina Bausch and many other dancers who transform everyday violence into choreography.

I am thinking of those writers who produce self-confessed fictional autobiogra-phies because they all recognize now that personal history is pure fiction.

I am thinking of artists like Joseph Beuys, Annette Messager, Christian Boltanski, Fromanger and their very specific ways of positioning themselves within the flux of social life.

I am thinking particularly of Marcel Duchamp who brought a urinal into the museum and presented it to the gaze of visitors as a piece of sculpture. By doing this he challenged the roots of our perception and made us realize that our reac-tion to a work of art depends on the context. In terms of my own interest in artistic creation and aesthetic practice there is a before-Duchamp and an after-Duchamp.

The encounter with Duchamp was highly influential in terms of transforming the way I look at things as a psychotherapist: re-situating what is commonplace and turning it into art.

. . . and I can think of many others too!

The aesthetics that inspires today's creators calls on us to live in the world in a better way. In other words, those of the modern art theorist Nicolas Bourriaud: "works of art no longer aim to create imagined or utopian realities but to form modes of existence or models of action within the here and now" (2011, p. 13).

Hence these creators show us the way to expanded modes and forms of contact.

2.   An Aesthetics of the Ephemeral

One of the most important contributions of the founders of gestalt therapy was to privilege temporality[2] alongside spatiality, even if metaphorically, as in the "topic" mode of thinking. Temporality is the here and now. ("Whatever exists is here and now. The past now as memory, nostalgia, regret, resentment, fantasy, legend, history. The future also exists here and now in the actual present as anticipation, planning, rehearsal expectation and hope, or dread and despair", Perls, 1989, p. 123). What happens within existing reality is the ongoing process of gestalt creation and destruction that we call *Gestaltung*, and the mutual transformation of figure and ground. It is the self-as-process, which emerges only through a creative engagement with difficult situations; it is the activating of the ego-functions of the self whenever it makes an identification or feels an alienation. Also in process are the constantly changing contact boundary, the oh-so-ephemeral emotions, the ways in which figure-formation is interrupted, the reference to field-experience, and so on.

In its refusal to fix experience into a definitive form, and to substitute one fixed *gestalt* for another, since we "never enter the same river twice" (Heraclitus) . . . our entire theory becomes focused on the aesthetics of the ephemeral. In contrast to other approaches which show an interest in structures, gestalt therapy always invites to a provisional dynamics.

Here again we can see a remarkable convergence with contemporary art.

Of course some artists follow tradition and carry on building cathedrals, or whatever the contemporary equivalent is, works intended to last. But the 20th century also saw the emergence of ephemeral art: installations, performances, works of art that are gradually destroyed by visitors and the actions of spectators, land art and all kinds of activities that take place within the landscape where nature gradually digests and reclaims them . . . I am also thinking of the wandering paths of dadaïst or surrealist art.

"Forms", in gestalt therapy, are no longer set forms but forms that move, and are, yet again: ephemeral. Goodman rephrases Von Weizsäcker's question: "What shape is water?" . . . Of course, water can only ever take the form of whatever contains it, for the time being . . .

The way we focus ourselves on what is felt, the pathic, our aiming that anything which in-sists may also ex-ist, shows we are concentrating on what is happening, on seeing whatever may happen as an event.

The ephemeral means taking advantage of the right moment, as Jankélévitch suggests in his philosophy of the occasion: seize things as they emerge.

Or according to the poet Henri Michaux (2004, p. 209), in our consciousness there are areas which are indefinite and discontinuities which are permanent.

So perhaps we may define consciousness-awareness as empathy with what is ephemeral, ephemeral feeling and perceiving.

3.   An Aesthetics of *Gestaltung*

"Form is the place where an organism meets its environment", wrote Von Weizsäcker. For Dewey, "Form is the way in which we shape and integrate our experiences" (1933, p. 184). It is form that selects and intensifies the spatial and temporal aspects of perception. The need for form and the experience of development are intimately linked: development is the organizing of experience over time, and form is what renders the nature of this organization explicit.

At this point I need to say a few words about what I refer to here as "form". I am not using the term in its metaphysical and platonic meaning but rather in the sense of "style", of "how" rather than "what". Form comes out of the endless transformation of the objective facticity of the real world into the subjective reality of the "creator".

In fact, as Laura Perls was at pains to point out, the gestalt therapist is more interested in the *Gestaltung* than the Gestalt. This *Gestaltung* was at the heart of Mondrian and Paul Klee's theories of art. In his Bauhaus teaching Klee wrote: "The theory of *Gestaltung* concerns the ways in which the Gestalt, the form is arrived at [. . .] The word *Gestaltung* is directly related to the concept [. . .] of a kind of mobility" (Klee, 1956, pp. 40–41 French translation 1964).

However it was above all Hans Prinzhorn (1922) who was to crystallize an artistic and psychiatric theory around the proposition that I have often had occasion to quote "We seek the meaning of every form that is formed by the act of formation itself".

Prinzhorn, following Klee, sees the need for self-expression as the basis of *Gestaltung*. These expressive movements differ from goal-oriented movements, they give flesh and blood to the psyche "so it is given to us in unmediated form within a lived participatory experience". They allow us to pass from living to form. These expressive movements come out of particular drives and needs:

– the drive to play (or to be active), and the impulse to adorn (to enrich the environment). These two impulses are enough to produce what I call scribbling. But further impulses are involved, namely:
– the tendency to reproduce (the drive to imitate) and the tendency to organize, both associated with the need for symbols. These enable the impulse towards *Gestaltung* to be directed towards the production of signs.

Prinzhorn added the need to communicate, but he does not appear to attach as much importance as we might wish to this aspect.

This drive towards *Gestaltung*, this desire to form, is close to Otto Rank's famous *will to form*, which had such a profound influence on the founders of the theory of gestalt therapy and formed the paradigm for their development of a theory of the self.

Henri Maldiney (1986), however, picked up what he saw as a mistake on the part of Prinzhorn: the latter actually located the origins of *Gestaltung* within the process of perception, whereas what *Gestaltung* gives us is not *gnosis*, or intellectual knowledge, but *pathos*, or sensory knowledge, that is, what is felt.

According to Maldiney, the origin of the *Gestaltung* should be situated in the ambit of feeling, and hence of the meaning of feeling. And here again we find aesthesis, aesthetics . . .

4.   An Aesthetics of Reworking

The notion of reworking, in the sense of repairing or mending, taken from Merleau-Ponty's notion of *reprise*, has a range of associations: I think of women of my grandmother's generation who used to spend hours darning socks, repairing them. This notion of repairing is familiar to psychotherapists, even though some may prefer to use metaphors like "weaving", "binding up", "knitting", or "folding/ unfolding" . . .

The material that is brought to the psychotherapeutic encounter becomes the object of reworking and mending. It is reworked and repaired, sometimes so that it can be let go of more easily. Take hold of, let go of . . .

Psychotherapy

> re-takes hold of a given, remakes it, restructures it, and pushes it further in a process which is simultaneously a recovery, a distortion, and a search which transforms the seeker. By going back to the beginning, by repeating and retaining, it also restarts, reshapes, repairs and recreates. The term "reworking" (*reprise*) always denotes an ambiguous gesture, a deliberate decision or intention to intervene in the pre-existent. Throughout the course of history, wherever people produce artifacts they also rework them.
>
> (Delcò, 2005, pp. 10–11)

When they were doing their mending, our grandmothers would start with the edges. And it is by starting at the edges of "what is" that growth, development and re-creation can happen. The edges, the margins, the leftovers, the footnotes, anything that has not been incorporated into the text of our experience and which can be reworked to form the body of a new text . . .

We might envisage the psychotherapeutic experience as one of centrality.

Just as gestalt therapy conceptualizes the self as decentralized at the point of contact, I believe that the psychotherapeutic experience takes place at the edge, at the boundary, and that the process of reconstruction starts from that edge.

5.   An Aesthetics of Standing Aside

Psychotherapists are often not where we expect to find them.

The same is true of creative artists. Otherwise they may still be artists, in the sense that art is their job, a job like any other, but they are not creative artists.

Creators are resisters because their work is always unique. The act of creation is an act of individuation within a context. The psychotherapist, just by being there as well as by any intervention he or she might make, is constantly introducing a gap between experience and its representation. Even their way of managing transference involves a gap: "the therapeutic meaning [of transference] is not that it is the same old story, but precisely that it is now differently worked through as a present adventure: the analyst not the same kind of parent", as Perls and Goodman wrote (1951/1994, p. 57).

"Stand out of the way" Goodman likes to say. "Stay aside!" Here he is adopting one of the precepts of Taoist philosophy.

. . . and the authorities clearly understand this only too well when they try to bring us in from the margins and turn us into the mental health police.

6.   . . . And This Brings Us to Interstices

Certain contemporary philosophers have borrowed this term "interstice" from Karl Marx, who applied it to communities of exchange which existed outside the framework of the capitalist economy because they did not adhere to its normal rules, particularly the pursuit of profit. The interstice introduces a space for relationships, a space which is partially integrated into the global system but where it is also possible to have different kinds of exchanges from those that operate within the system. (It is difficult not to be reminded here of the eco-niche, or ecological niche so dear to Goodman.)

As I said before, the creator is a resister because his or her work is unique. If art is "the invention of possible ways of being" (Nietzsche), then the act of creation is an act of differentiation, of individuation within a context, as Otto Rank showed so well. The creator opens up interstices and fissures in any ordered and logically organized system. So the creator is not on the outside: Otto Rank also wrote in *Art and the Artist* (a work that is "beyond praise", according to Perls, Hefferline and Goodman) that "the artist creates art and at the same time uses art in order to create" (Rank, 1932, p. 34).

For me "interstice" is associated with a number of other concepts, ideas and actions: particularly the syncope which interrupts the smooth rhythm of breathing, or the fissure that appears in the heart of our certainties and makes them crumble, and others too.

7.   An Aesthetics of the Situation

These aesthetic ingredients constitute an aesthetic of the situation.

Psychotherapeutic encounters consist in a succession of contacts, and each of these encounters constitutes a situation. "Our existence is embodied in a succession of constantly developing and changing situations that come upon us unexpectedly. To be situated, to be an integral part of a situation, is tantamount to existing as a human being" (Buijtendijk, 1954).[3]

"The structure of a situation is the internal coherence of its form and content", claims Goodman (Perls, Hefferline and Goodman, 1951/1994, p. 114). So it is both our function and our responsibility to help define the situation in such a way that we can apply aesthetic criteria when structuring the experience. This is why I introduced the concept of affordance in my earlier work, a term borrowed from Gibson, a disciple of Lewin. The idea of affordance is that the environment presents certain features that are capable of attracting me (me, but not necessarily you!) and that these partially structure my desire. So, since needs and desires are always a function of the total situation (what we refer to as, following Goodman "the *id* of the situation", the question is, how may I best structure my patient's environment, of which I am part, in the here and now, so that I can offer him or her forms that are attractive, forms that will encourage movement and creation? . . .

In contemporary art, a number of creative artists present what are essentially situations. Of course, Debord and the situationist movement come to mind here, but there are also all those artistic practices that I mentioned in relation to the ephemeral, since all situations are by definition ephemeral.

Contemporary aesthetics enables us to overcome the separation between the production of material goods (*poiesis*) and the production of the self through individual creative practice (*praxis*), and to make praxis equivalent to poiesis.

To create also means to create oneself. The creation of the self and the creation of a work of art are no longer two separate processes.

This aesthetic definition of the situation gives rise to the aesthetics of commitment that Laura Perls, Michael Miller and Dan Bloom have spoken of so extensively.

In her last work, *Commitment*, Laura Perls takes the example of the film *Woman in the Dunes* and writes:

> The man takes responsibility for the *consequences* of his own creative activities. He himself has opened the trap of his own personal limitations, the conditioned habits, attitudes and prejudices, the fixed *gestalten* of his former previous lives. By accepting and coping with "what is", he transforms and transcends the situation and achieves true freedom.

> (Perls, 1989, p. 191)

This aesthetic is summed up by Laura Perls thus: "Living with uncertainty without anxiety."

8.   The Aesthetic Paradigm in Psychotherapy

I have found a certain convergence with the aesthetic approach of gestalt therapy in the work of Félix Guattari. He believes that this paradigm can enrich psychiatric practice and free it from dependence on a "scientistic superego" which sets practice in stone. "My perspective involves shifting the human and social sciences from scientific paradigms towards ethico-aesthetic paradigms" (Guattari, 1995, p. 11).

Guattari's philosophical project, which is to be found scattered throughout his writings, includes this concern: "What is important is to know if a work leads effectively to a mutant production of enunciation" (Guattari, 1995, p. 19). The psychotherapist shares this concern and expresses it in the same terms: the important thing is to see whether a particular psychotherapeutic intervention will help bring about a *mutant production of enunciation*. Both art and psychotherapy (Guattari preferred to speak of psychoanalysis) are potential aesthetics, they are two modalities of producing subjectivity, a never-ending process. Psychotherapy and artistic practice are two of the most important ways of doing this.

I say "are" but it would probably be more accurate to say "may be" because I am aware that certain so-called psychotherapeutic practices may be about control, and some artistic practice is just about producing consumer objects. "Psychotherapy" is not the only way of altering minds!

For example, Félix Guattari wrote, in *Chaosmosis*: "One creates new modalities of subjectivity in the same way that an artist creates new forms from the palette [of available materials]" (1995, p. 7). Guattari as well, in his own way, tries to de-territorialize subjectivity, to de-tach it from the subject, just as Paul Goodman, several decades previously, had striven to delocalize the psyche and hence the self, as I was able to show in previous works. For Guattari, as for gestalt therapists like ourselves, subjectivity can only be defined in relation to another subjectivity. It cannot exist on its own, nor can it form the basis of the subject's existence. Subjectivity for him is the totality of the relationships formed between the individual and the vectors of subjectivation, both human and non-human, that he or she encounters. These views, although emerging from a different conceptual framework, are the basic ideas underlying gestalt therapy: contact as primary experience, the self as something active and self-aware.

> He goes in search of whatever is breaking down, escaping, and allowing us to creep inside it, outside the dominant redundancies. He is prepared to root around in all kinds of garbage – society's garbage, philosophical garbage, all kinds of conceptual garbage – to find a way out, to break free of our bogged-down perceptions and affections, and to produce mutant percepts and affects [. . .] To produce a way of feeling that will bring about mutations in the sphere of the infinite . . .
>
> (Guattari in Zahm, 1994, p. 8).

Is Guattari referring here to the artist or to the psychotherapist?

The artist, like the psychotherapist, is someone who "works on meanings" rather than a creator dependent on divine inspiration. The artist is even someone who: "works on fissures in subjectivity", to use Guattari's particularly apposite phrase.

"Artists are like knights errant, the Don Quixotes of a certain type of subjectivation in a dying age of chivalry" (Guattari in Zahm, 1994, p. 5).

In conclusion, I will quote the words of Monica Alvim, a Brazilian colleague and friend, whose work combines the challenges posed by both aesthetics and psychotherapy in a common project: that of reconciliation. Reconciliation between art that launches an all-out attack on convention, and the public. Reconciliation between a life-work and the person who lives and creates it, with the help of the therapist.

> Looking at this life-work through the eyes of aesthetic experience, and transforming into an aesthetic object means that its creator can be reconciled with his or her own creation, [. . .] and thus with the world. Even, if need be, by using shock tactics and having the courage to transgress the given.
>
> (Alvim, 2004, p. 10)

Context: From my earliest encounters with gestalt therapy, I was impressed not only by the frequent use of artistic mediators to foster creativity in the course of therapy, but also and above all by the concepts that enabled me to draw on aesthetics, a branch of philosophy, in preference to pathology or the medical paradigm. This reflection and the different ways in which the concept of form, for example, is expressed, have never ceased to nourish my practice.

This chapter is the opening lecture of the conference I organized on this theme in Bordeaux in 2006, which led to the publication of J.-M. Robine (ed.), La psychothérapie comme esthétique, L'exprimerie, 2006.

Notes

1 In the original French there is a play on words which it is not possible to render in English: "pré" means both "pre-" or "before" and "meadow" [Translator's note.]
2 Robine (2004), p. 49 and pp. 103 and following.
3 Buijtendijk F.J.J. (1954). *Foreword* to the *Situation Review*, vol. 1, cited by Wollants (2005). [Unfortunately there will be no further issues of this review.]

Chapter 13

Therapy of Forms and Forms of Therapy

Therapy supposedly concerns the "deepest", most essential parts of the human being. The ancients gave the name "soul" to this deepest, most essential part of us, and to free it from the religious connotation accumulated by this term over the centuries, another name was assigned to this notion in the nineteenth century: the psyche. This concept, borrowed from ancient Greek, was almost immediately accompanied by the birth of a new discipline, to which it helped provide a name: psychotherapy.

The combination of these two concepts ("psyche" and "therapy") leaves the nature of their relationship rather vague: a therapy *of* the psyche? Or therapy *through* the psyche? Comparing it to other "therapies" does little to resolve the ambiguity: chemotherapy, mesotherapy, balneotherapy, hippotherapy, hypnotherapy, art therapy, dance therapy, play therapy, etc. all designate the means and methods according to which the therapy operates.

However, general dictionaries usually define psychotherapy as an intervention carried out on the psyche – a therapy *of* the psyche – although they occasionally add that this takes place through *psycho*logical processes. Psychotherapy could thus be defined as a therapy of the psyche through the psyche, just as physical therapy could be defined as a therapy *of* movement *through* movement.

It is therefore possible that the means and the end merge together – that the journey is also the destination; the process is also the target.

1. A Relocation of the Psyche

Phenomenology paved the way by urging us to abandon the surface/depth distinction upon which contemporary psychology and psychoanalysis are based. Since this involves spatializing experience, Lacan used topological objects to challenge our representations of experience. A Möbius strip, for example, materializes how the front side may be found on the reverse side, just as the conscious may be found in the unconscious and the unconscious in the conscious, the depths on the surface and vice versa, uninterrupted.

Gestalt therapy, which was grounded in psychoanalysis thanks to its founder F. Perls, also took shape under the influence of Paul Goodman, an American

DOI: 10.4324/9781003515760-16

thinker who was familiar with the ideas developed by American pragmatists and phenomenologists. Starting from the traditional "psyche-based" model – which, whether he liked it or not, is relatively consistent with Perls' thought process and background – by incorporating Goodman's contribution, it is possible to continue and extend their proposals, in particular by laying out certain proposals scattered throughout their joint work that have long gone overlooked.

Their proposal represents a radical paradigm shift, with "radical" being used in the fullest sense of the term, i.e. "concerning the roots": "contact [. . .] is the simplest and first reality".

This premise allows them to open their manifesto with these words, which are the direct result of it: "Experience occurs at the boundary between the organism and its environment, primarily the skin surface and the other organs of sensory and motor response" (Perls, Hefferline and Goodman, 1951/1994, p. 49). It involves rehabilitating the "surface" and relocating experience, which is no longer buried in the "depths of being", but instead in the "in between": between the organism and the human and non-human environment. Before the word "psyche" designated the soul, it meant the breath of life; in this theory, it becomes contact once again, since breathing is the first contact a human has with the world, and it remains the most fundamental contact: our essential link to the world.

The authors immediately continue: "Experience is the function of this boundary, and psychologically what is real are the 'whole' configurations of this functioning, some meaning being achieved, some action completed" (Perls, Hefferline and Goodman, 1951/1994, p. 49).

The construction of meaning and implementation of actions are not theorized as belonging to a function of the psyche, but rather as an operation of "in between": the operation that connects the subject and its environment. This is what we call "field perspective", with the field itself being defined as a unit composed of a given organism and its environment. This perspective thus distinguishes itself from the traditional individualistic, intrapsychic perspective to make up a whole new paradigm which both opposes and encompasses what came before.

2.   What Happens in This "In Between"?

The *in between* is the boundary area where contact operations unfold: consciousness, motor response, actions, sensations and emotions, thoughts and dialogues: ". . . every kind of living relation that occurs at the boundary in the interaction of the organism and environment" (Perls, Hefferline and Goodman, 1951/1994, p. 52).

Although the word "contact" is commonly used in everyday language, in gestalt therapy it refers to a complex operation composed of at least two essential ingredients: consciousness and motor activity. It should be noted that this consciousness may be nothing but an immediate, implicit awareness, and motor activity may be as rudimentary as looking towards something, listening in on something, modifying one's breathing, etc.

This awareness – or *intentionality*, as we might say, drawing upon the work of Husserl – constructs figure/ground relations: it brings elements to the foreground, selecting extracts among the range of possibilities to make them into signifiers. They are signifiers by virtue of the investment they receive from the activity of awareness, and signifiers in the relationship established with the background elements that give depth, salience and direction of meaning to this figure of interest.

Contact is constructing meaning. Contact is constructing a form. Contact is being present in a situation. And since every situation is new, even though it may have certain similarities with previously encountered situations, each contact will involve both adaptation and creation. The forms that creative adaptation may take in a given situation are manifold, but the forms that may be taken by the interruptions, distortions, inhibitions or fixations of this creative adjustment activity are limited, and these inflections of experience are what will guide the therapeutic procedure.

3.   The Therapy of Forms

Therapy is thus no longer defined as an analysis of the psyche (*psycho-analysis*) or as a therapy of the psyche (*psycho-therapy*) but as an analysis and therapy of *gestalts*: of these forms, these figure/ground relations that may be defective, frozen, dysfunctional or inconsistent. The analysis of these gestalts thus leads to a *therapy of the gestalt*, i.e. a therapy of forms, which will work by intervening in the formation of these forms, otherwise known as *Gestaltung*.

These forms are creative adjustments that allow or require contact with the environment. As I mentioned above ("It is therefore possible that the means and the end merge together – that the journey is also the destination; the process is also the target"), creative adjustment is both the objective in therapy and the means to achieve it.

The concept of creative adjustment seems to be the paradoxical juxtaposition of two concepts that pull the experience in opposite directions. Through adjustment, the individual adapts to her environment: she transforms herself (or is transformed) by the environment in order to correspond to its opportunities and benefit from these affordances.[1] The environment contains possibilities, a medium and substances that give form to objects and other living things, and "offer" the animal and the human animal different interaction possibilities. Gibson uses the term *affordances* to describe interaction possibilities offered to the animal by its environment. If I am tired of standing up and my environment places a chair in my visual field (*affordance*), in order to sit down I will have to adapt the shape of my body to that of the chair, adjusting my posture to this resource and its constraints and limitations.

Historically, in the late forties – when Perls and Goodman were setting the foundations for gestalt therapy – psychotherapy and psychoanalysis were heavily criticized for placing too much emphasis on adapting the individual to society. Based on the question of what meaning there may be in aiming to adapt the individual to a pathogenic society – although at least a minimal level of adaptation is necessary – the authors associated the term "creative" with the concept of adjustment. The adjective "creative", in my opinion, should be understood in an active rather than a passive sense. The authors' work – especially Goodman's – shows that adaptation is not limited to a *potential* (since "creative" and "creativity" refer to the possibility of something culminating in a creation) – instead, it must be truly *transformative*. In and through the same act of creative adjustment, my contact with the world transforms me and I transform the world. This mutual transformation need not be seen as utopian or wishful thinking: it can be demonstrated by forms of contact with the world as basic as breathing. When I inhale, I am transformed; when I exhale, the world is transformed.

If therapy is treated as a therapy of the process of constructing/deconstructing *gestalts*, it is the "how" of the experience – much more than the "what" and even more than the "why" – that the protagonists will focus on: both patient and therapist. The form will appear in the way the person does what he or she does, not in what he or she does or why he or she does it. If we take the example of artistic creation, the fact that Cézanne chose to paint a few apples is not what interests us about his work, nor do we seek to discover why he painted apples and not cherries, flowers, utensils or portraits; instead, we are interested in how he treats his subject, his creative process, his approach – in short, by the act of taking form.

4. What Is a Form?

Since the time of Heraclitus, there has been an opposition between what flows and what remains: between the ephemeral and the stable. Since the beginnings of philosophy and of science – which for the Greeks were not separate ventures – what is stable has been given the name "form".

The concept of form was then joined by other words: structure, pattern, figure, gestalt, appearance, mould, etc.

Biology, chemistry, mathematics and physics make use of this concept, as do linguistics, psychology, philosophy and aesthetics. However, for all these disciplines, beyond the unavoidable variations related to their subjects, form refers to a configuration of parts seen as a whole, and this whole is what defines the parts and renders them interdependent.

This relatively stable concept of form is joined by notions of consistency and coherence, and even of order, harmony and balance.

Among the many Greek words that have been translated as "form", we should of course remember *morphè*, which produced a number of variations that will be of interest to the therapist: morphogenesis, morphology, anamorphosis, metamorphosis, hylomorphism and even Morpheus, the god of sleep and of the dreams that inspire many created forms.

However, this specific arrangement between the parts and the whole – the spatial organization of things in motion – was referred to by another word: *rhythm*.

This differentiation leads us to anchor this concept in the temporal and dynamic dimension, and to free it from the fixity in which it may be trapped.

We should not forget *eidos*, which became an "idea" but initially referred to the form – as opposed to the material – of the body or a thing; it was later used in poetry to refer to the person him- or herself, and finally as the form of something present in the mind: thus, "the idea". Knowing something is contemplating its form.

It took more than two millennia for the concept of form – or its equivalent, the gestalt – to return once again to the centre of a system of thought, albeit in a slightly different way. Gestalt *psychology* first examined the various factors that promote the organization of the perceptual field, before becoming gestalt *theory* in order to extend certain discoveries made in the realm of perception to other phenomena. With gestalt theory, the primary experience of awareness is highlighted because the perceiving form (the phenomenal pattern) is what unifies the perceived contents.

At the end of the nineteenth century and the first half of the twentieth, gestalt theorists were able to highlight the characteristics of the *Gestalt*, a German word usually translated as "form" although the two concepts do not completely overlap; they then expanded their domain to assert, for example, a number of principles deriving from it. The concept of form was separated from its visual and superficial connotations to be treated as a relative configuration of similar or related items. From this perspective, gestalt theorists argue that the interaction between the individual and the situation (dynamic field) is what determines the experience and the construction of forms, and not only the behaviour, drives, external stimuli or personality traits of a given individual.

5.   Form or Formation of Forms?

Despite the insistence of certain authors, the concept of form is often connected to the idea of fixity and stability. Psychologists and psychotherapists are much more concerned with dynamic, temporary or metastable forms, since they are alive, than they are by static (and therefore dead) forms. This is why writers like Prinzhorn built their theory of the relationship between creation and pathology on the concept of *Gestaltung* and not on *gestalt*. Here, the concept of *the formation of forms* is equivalent to that of *Gestaltung*.

In *Gestaltung*, emphasis is placed on the process: the movement of taking shape. Creative expression therapies focus more on the process than on the object created, while in gestalt therapy, the sequence of construction/deconstruction of the figure/ground relation in the present moment serves as a guide. Understanding the work of art is phenomenologically oriented toward the process as well, far from being a psychoanalytic interpretation of manifest and latent content. "We seek the meaning of each form formed in the act of formation itself", wrote Prinzhorn. Henri Maldiney[2] followed the same approach throughout the part of his work dedicated to art. Gestalt therapists draw on this approach to creation to guide their patients in constructing meaning based on the formation of their everyday forms of contact.

In other words, for the psychologist or psychotherapist, a form cannot be separated from its own dynamics. P. Quéau (1989) beautifully connects the two concepts as follows: "Forms and forces are two distinct faces of the same reality. A form is a fixed force; a force is a fluid form. Forces in action are potential forms, and vice versa" (p. 301).

Moreover, as we know from the aforementioned gestalt theorists, a form is given meaning both *in* and *by* the situation. Gestalt therapists would phrase it as "in contact". In his interview with Emile Noël, René Thom takes the example of a magnifying glass: a simple piece of glass which, when placed in a specific situation, can ignite a piece of paper by putting it in "contact" with sunlight. He also cites the example of a propeller turning in the wind which provides a stream of energy. Although these objects or forms may appear lifeless because they are immobilized, trapped within the boundaries of their own edges, might we say that they are capable of becoming metastable and "alive" once again when placed in specific situations and appropriate types of contact? A field perspective is indeed the only perspective that allows us to free ourselves from the isolationist vision of form because it connects force and form.

This conception of form is of paramount importance to psychotherapists, especially those who defined themselves as *gestalt therapists*, i.e. therapists of forms (meaning: that each of us has been able to give to our existence). To illustrate this perspective, I would like to briefly mention two examples of the use of a way of thinking that could be based on form: emotions and symptoms.

6.   A Formation of Forms: Emotion

A vast number of philosophical, phenomenological, ethological, psychological, anthropological, psychotherapeutic, sociological and other studies have been conducted on emotions, and I have no intention of calling these studies into question or contradicting them. I would just like to mention some of the issues raised by my practice of psychotherapy. What I object to, however, among the usual theories of emotion is the assumption that emotion can be a primary phenomenon, in the sense that there is no other experience preceding it.

According to the culture, context and relational situations involved, the "emotional" experience can take different *forms*. Certainly, the word "emotion" comes from the Latin *ex-movere* which means "to set in motion", but it also contains the "ex-" prefix that indicates the *ex*ternalization of that setting in motion. In my view, what comes first is indeed this "setting in motion" *within* the body, which is initially only a feeling – a "pre-" experience: preverbal, pre-emotional, pre-significant. This is about the "vague and confused", to use Minkowski's terms. This bodily experience cannot last long without meaning or form: it is therefore given form both *in* and *by* contact, in a given situation. I am assuming that emotion is a *form* produced by contact and the situation, not the production of a specific subject. Considered in this light, emotion is an indicator of the situation: it is a field phenomenon and, as such, it reveals something about the state of the field at a given moment (i.e. of a specific organism in contact with its environment). Emotion provides information on the *state* of the organism confronted with the *state* of its environment, and thus also provides information on the characteristics of the environment in the immediacy of the situation.

Therapists often hear patients describe their pent-up anger or their unexpressed sadness. Patients can usually even locate "the emotion" within their bodies, deep down in their guts. If they are encouraged and supported in expressing this "anger", patients may utter or shout a few angry words which quickly turn into sobs. My hypothesis is that the relational and situational context, including the therapist's personality, favours one form being taken over another. As is the case in the epigenesis of the subject, a child may be explicitly asked to give another form to his feelings because the parent cannot accept the form used by the child: "Big boys don't cry!" So what does the child do in this case? He uses another form that is available and supported by his family and friends at that moment in time, such an aggressive form (since, as we know, *all* boys enjoy being aggressive and only girls cry!).

Yet the patient claims to experience anger that twists his stomach and that he cannot externalize. My reading is a pragmatic one, and not necessarily the same as the patient's: I implicitly assume that he is having a raw bodily experience (sensation, feeling, affect) but that this experience cannot remain formless and unverbalized. Based on the self's personality function – i.e. the system of self-representations drawn from prior experiences – the person uses the term "anger" for what it would probably be more accurate to describe as follows: "I feel such and such a sensation in my body and I *imagine* that if I were to externalize it – if I placed it in contact with the world – it would be in the form of anger!" In many cases, this may be what will happen if the situation permits it, because the subject is looking for confirmation in the representations he has of himself, so he reproduces what he knows how to do. In doing so, he locks himself inside the reproduction of a form and no longer creates contact, in relation to the elements of the situation which always involve aspects that are unknown and new.

As a gestalt therapist, I know that the emotions present in an encounter – both the client's and my own – represent one of the possible forms of the organization of the current experience. If it is approached as a *form* of experience, an emotion is an invitation to continue exploring in order to access the *experience*, and to consider whether this form is creation, creative adjustment and a choice from among the possible choices, rather than fixation, habit, routine or second nature. If it turns out that this form is a repetition of a fixed form, the question arises of how to re-access the possibilities of creating adjusted, creative forms.

7.   Another Example of Form: The Symptom

When placed in situations of intense difficulty, the individual is required to construct an appropriate response that takes the parameters of the situation into account. His response involves an overall configuration which includes elements that may be physical, bodily, affective, emotional, representational, motor-related, mental, relational, etc. This form, created in a given context, is a creative adjustment in that it attempts to resolve the problem as best it can using the means at hand: i.e. the materials available, affordances, codes and other resources.

This configuration is appropriate, while occasionally uneconomical for its creator, and it has a function – even a dual function, as has been clearly shown by generations of psychologists interested in humans beyond their cognitive and behavioural components. This configuration indicates that there is a problem that it simultaneously hides *and*, through this form, tries to solve.

In a number of cases, establishing this overall configuration does actually allow the problem to be dissolved or resolved. In this case, the pattern extinguishes itself, sometimes without the subject even being aware of it.

In other cases in which attempts are made to solve the initial problem, the pattern itself may become the problem, as may be the case with obsessional rituals, addictions and many other "symptoms". The establishment of this form, which is adapted or relatively adapted to a given context, becomes obsolete through its temporal and spatial decontextualization, thereby losing most of its function. To return to the image of the propeller used by René Thom, this form was created by a given subject and adapted to provide him with energy using the force of the wind when it was necessary, but it is now being kept in a glass case that he carries around with him, regardless of where he goes and what he does.

If we accept the working hypothesis that consists in addressing the symptom as a form, thus aligning ourselves with the views of Otto Rank, who described the neurotic as a "failed artist", the therapeutic task can be approached in a perceptibly different manner (and when I say "perceptibly different", I am aware that all the "perceptible" components of this creation can thus be taken into account). This conception dates back to the early twentieth century, and it would be fruitful to extend its analysis to address symptoms as a style, not only as a disease.[3]

The symptom is a form: one which has been adapted and is appropriate to a situation, a context and/or a relational system – a form of contact. It is most definitely an inflected form, suffering and generating suffering, because it is often full of clumsy missteps. This form externalizes, expresses and says something to someone. It is there for a reason, even if it is not always easy to understand its origin, its choice, its meaning, its function, its grammar or its lexicon. If the form's adjustment characteristics are obsolete, the therapeutic task can be designed around the construction of new forms, with the destruction of fixed forms in favour of fluid, metastable forms which to the fullest extent possible should be more economical, better suited to the situation and more efficient in their functioning. Incidentally, this is one reason why many psychotherapists – or many gestalt therapists, at least – attach so much importance to the development of creative processes, and to this end, as part of the healing process, implement the use of artistic mediators: they provide a training ground or test site for the creation of forms of existence.

8.   Conclusion: Psychotherapy as an Aesthetic

Therapists who dare to place the concept of form at the centre of their approach to human experience thereby remove the concept of disease from its position as the essential paradigm. Their type of psychotherapy is characterized not only by a scientific approach[4] but first and foremost by an aesthetic approach, i.e. one that is anchored in a philosophical approach based on the sensitive qualities of form. Health is thus addressed "as the ability to create forms that are adapted to situations, and pathology as the loss of this potential which leads to reliance on fixed forms which are inadequate or obsolete – scribbling" (Robine, 2006a).

This certainly does not come with the corollary that psychotherapists have to define or identify themselves as artists, contrary to the claims of some in an attempt to justify their refusal to acquire the techniques and knowledge required for such an exercise. While working with a therapist, the patient is able to become a kind of artist – a creator of his or her existence: that is to say, forms that are flexible, significant, limited, coherent, articulate, adjusted, creative and consistent. In the words of Isadore From, a member of the group that founded gestalt therapy, the goal of psychotherapy is to help clients "transform their speech into poetry and their walk into dance" – work that involves the formation of forms.

Context: Before I came across gestalt therapy, I had been practising "expression therapy", which was undoubtedly the "royal road" that led me to it. I was therefore delighted to have the opportunity to address both expression therapists ("Is there anyone out there?" in a previous book) and art therapists with this lecture. This text was published in Art et thérapie, *no. 102/103, in 2009.*

Notes

1   Noun created from the verb "to afford". The psychology of Gibson (a student of Kurt Lewin, who was himself an advocate of field perspective in psychology and social psychology) was developed based on the concept of affordance. Gibson uses the term *affordances* to refer to the possibilities of interaction offered to the animal by its environment (Gibson, 1979).

2   See, for example: Maldiney (1985; 1993; 1997) and his works on Ponge, Tal-Coat, Bazaine, etc.

3   See, for example, Steiner and Moralès (1997).

4   The current trend, with the complicity of the public authorities, encourages the so-called "scientific" approach to psychotherapy. It has only succeeded in creating a temporarily profitable illusion; a wide range of studies have clearly shown that the supposedly scientific nature of this approach was nothing but an illusion: the "scientistic" mask of corporatist lobbying.

Chapter 14

"Structions"

As an introduction to what I'd like to contribute to our thinking on the topic of "the construction/destruction of *gestalts*", I'd like to mention two personal memories related to this subject. The first concerns Isadore From and took place around 1980. At one of my training sessions with him, I asked him a question, roughly as follows:

> Since most patients come to us with unfinished, unassimilated, poorly integrated situations, couldn't we say that therapeutic work begins much more often with post-contact work than with fore-contact, since the post-contact phase is described as a phase of integrating experience and assimilation, and involves relaunching this interrupted assimilation?

Isadore, who was a little surprised by my question, showed me that this wasn't the case because even though we were working on stuck, blocked, unfinished situations, we still had no choice but to start with fore-contact since these terms refer to the dynamics of the construction/destruction of a figure in the present moment, even if this involves supposedly old material.

The other story took place at about the same time. I was enrolled in a training seminar with Virginia Satir, a major figure in family therapy who was quite close to gestalt therapy through her acquaintance with Perls during the years they both spent at Esalen. On therapeutic work, she essentially said, "Remember that therapeutic work is certainly not about removing or withdrawing anything whatsoever from the patient, even his symptoms or suffering. Therapeutic work is about giving him something more: letting him leave with something extra so that, thanks to this "something more", he no longer needs a number of elements of his experience and his fixations: he can get rid of them without even having to consciously focus on it". Something more and not something less; we could therefore say, using our contemporary vocabulary, something to construct much more than something to destroy.

This leads me to ask myself (and ourselves) the following question: in psychotherapy, aren't constructing and destroying basically one and the same operation? Unlike the metaphor of architecture used by Jacques Blaize (2005) that evokes the

DOI: 10.4324/9781003515760-17

construction of a house – a situation involving physical materials – in the psycho-logical realm, aren't construction and destruction a single, simultaneous operation?

When I first started looking into the question of the "construction/destruction" of a *gestalt*, one of my first thoughts, in the form of an amused question, was oriented towards the words involved. Why are words like de*struction*, con*struction*, in*struction*, decon*struction*, ob*struction*, etc. always compound words (de-struct, con-struct, in-struct, etc.)? What is this "struct" to which we always add a prefix? Is there an operation called "struction"? No! It doesn't exist in English, but in its Latin root *struere* the verb exists and means "to build or pile up" into a structure. It is also worth noting that construction, destruction, etc. have the same etymology as "structure".

It is therefore interesting to remark that, in our language, "struct" only exists in compound forms. Could *in*struct perhaps consist of depositing layers inside the other? Does *con*struct mean "struct with"? Whether we work *with* materials or *with* others, there is always a "with" involved . . . which suggests that we cannot "struct" alone. If there is always a "with", the concept of "co-construction" is a stuttering redundancy! The question then arises: why, in recent years, have we been led to use and abuse this concept of co-construction? This concept was hardly ever used ten or twenty years ago. My theory is that the surge in our use of the concept of co-construction essentially arose as a defence related to the position of power we could have in the therapeutic relationship. Wanting to focus on the "co-" probably reflects an attempt to partake in the egalitarian myth: we're doing it "together"; it isn't about one of us working *on* the other. This is only a hypothesis, but perhaps this co-construction neologism offers us a certain blindness: a way to deny our position of expertise or our position of power, and at some point we will have to return to this question of expertise and power.

Some of you have probably read Rupert Sheldrake's work on morphogenetic fields: how the field itself can generate forms. One example he cites comes to mind: that of termites building their mounds, these huge arches that can be found in certain deserts. Millions or even billions of insects are involved in building the mound together. Termites obviously have less elaborate brains than humans, and they have no memory or programming telling them what type of work they need to do, since there are countless possibilities depending on the place they occupy in constructing the mound. They cannot possibly have such complex, differenti-ated cell programming that billions of possible commands could be hard-wired into them to indicate exactly what they should do according to the role they play. You can imagine how limited a termite's visual field must be while constructing a mound that may be up to thirty feet high . . . and yet each termite knows exactly what it has to do according to its role in constructing the mound. This means that the field – the situation – is what structures and governs its work.

Don't we find something similar in the therapeutic relationship? We occupy a certain position, and that position dictates our function; naturally, our function and position is not the same as our client's. For me, this "co-" goes too far in implying a pseudo-egalitarian principle, while we have neither the same task nor the same function.

I would now like address the concepts of deconstruction and destruction. What might we have to destroy? What might we have to deconstruct together (to use the vocabulary that I was just critiquing a moment ago)?

1.   Deconstruction *in* Therapy

Constructing what? Deconstructing what? Can we deconstruct for the other, or do we deconstruct the other? Can we change the other? What I believe we can deconstruct (or at least contribute to deconstructing) is essentially a system of representation: these fixed forms that make us suffer. They are the patterns of meaning that we assign to the events we experience. You may object that there is no event without meaning, but I don't believe it is that simple. A few years ago, I mentioned Wittgenstein's well-known phrase stating that the limits of our experience are the limits of our language. It does not seem so obvious to me that we should limit our experience to what can be put into words. I believe that there are vast swathes of our experience of which we are "aware", or of which we may have some memory in the realm of the implicit. If indeed we limit our experience to our language and therefore to the system of representations that has been developed and constructed, I think that by doing so we limit our therapeutic resources.

So deconstruction: the deconstruction of systems of representation, outdated systems of contact, relationships, choices, choices without choices, choices based on introjects . . . Deconstruction! I like the word Max Pagès used a few years ago, "amalgams": deconstructing amalgams, these representational modalities that stick together an event, an affect, a representation, bodily sensations, the movement of an action . . . collages that solidify over time. Another author who developed a relatively similar idea is Vasilis Siomopoulos, an American psychiatrist who, in his treatise on psychopathology, called it the *object-affect-Gestalt*, which also refers to these collages or amalgams that occur and glue together all the emotional elements, bodily elements, relational objects, etc. I think that, in a way, one of the operations of psychotherapy lies in blowing up these amalgams. This is not to say that we have explosives or that we should work in the register of violence or of an attack on defence systems, but that simply employing (challenging, explaining, unfolding, etc.) a certain number of obvious truths – the sort of obvious truths that lead us to confluence, since we are in confluence with everything that seems obvious – is undoubtedly a milestone in the work of deconstruction.

I've noticed that in my therapeutic work, especially in recent years, virtually not a session goes by without the patient, student or supervisee – the person with whom work is being done – encountering confusion, vagueness, bewilderment, destabilization or chaos: for a moment, all their representations are no longer accessible; they temporarily lose sign of all their reference points. Obviously, this can cause anxiety for the client as well as the therapist. At such moments, the therapist may quickly seize the opportunity to spoonfeed a good introject, a good performance, or any other "good" way to reduce anxiety.

However, I find that such moments of anxiety are the most exceptional because, since we cannot cling to what is already known, the psychotherapist's alertness may cause the patient to open his eyes to the now. The now contains novelty; it is even the *only* "place" where there is novelty and the unknown. As a result, the breakdown of fixed forms, disintegration of obsolete forms and opening up to the now are put to "work" to allow the patient to construct his experience by making room for the now.

For a long time, I hated the use of the term "work" in therapy (as in "We need to work on this or that"), until I came across an author – Lévinas, I believe – who essentially said "I use the word 'work' in the sense that we use when talking about working a piece of wood: it twists, it cracks, it contracts or expands, and it changes". I like this metaphor for therapeutic work.

Putting the characteristics of the encounter back to work also means deconstructing individualistic belief in therapy. As you may know, gestalt therapy was probably one of the first therapeutic movements to have incorporated the concept of self. In my opinion, this component was introduced by George Herbert Mead, author of the famous book *Mind, Self and Society*. Although he is never mentioned by Perls and Goodman, it is likely that Mead indirectly contributed a great deal to Goodman's development of the theory of self. When Perls and Goodman mentioned the models that had helped them develop the theory of self, they cited Otto Rank for the reference to the artist in a creative situation, but did not mention George Herbert Mead, who had developed his own theory of self based on observations of children at play, even though Goodman used these two paradigms to construct his theory of self. Furthermore, George Herbert Mead, with his intellectual movement that took on the name "symbolic interactionism", introduced probably the clearest, most powerful iteration of the idea that belief should be dissolved in individualism. To quote a sentence from Mead, "No hard-and-fast line can be drawn between our own selves and the selves of others, since our own selves exist and enter as such into our experience only in so far as the selves of others exist and enter as such into our experience also."

All these beliefs that are to be broken down or deconstructed are supported by the constructions of realities by individuals, and these realities are maintained by social interactions and, in turn, these social interactions confirm the beliefs that originate in the realm of the social, and so goes the system. From the moment we open our eyes on the now in therapy, I think something can start working.

2.   Deconstruction *as* Therapy

Frank Staemmler wrote a book called *Cultivated Uncertainty*; Jacques Blaize wrote one called *Ne plus savoir* ("No longer knowing"). These themes refer to the practice of therapy and implicitly call for the deconstruction of something. I myself often discuss the practice of "offsetting" (not placing ourselves where the patient expects us to be); we also talk about the questioning of language, of the non-verbal, of beliefs, etc. This takes place *in* therapy but also *as* therapy!

I don't think there needs to be a distinction between knowing and acting: knowledge becomes an action from which meaning emerges through the coordination or confrontation between the therapist's beliefs and those of the patient. The shock of the patient's world map colliding with that of the therapist is in itself a deconstruction for each person involved.

We should be aware that asking a question of course involves requesting information, but at the same time it also involves providing information. When I ask the brilliant, original, essential, idiosyncratic question that every good Gestalt therapist asks his or her patient – "What are you feeling now?" – I'm *saying* something to my patient; I'm telling him, "Feelings are the foundation of all experience; feelings are what's important to me!", and so on. Every question I ask serves as a model; each one provides information on my values, my convictions and my structures.

Can therapy simultaneously deconstruct something and reconstruct it with a more critical, dialectical meaning? Forms can be extremely varied. A few weeks ago, I had an individual supervision session with a therapist whom I've been coaching for ten or twelve years. He told me about a session with an extremely violent nine-year-old child who'd been rejected by all the other therapists because he was even aggressive towards them. The therapist conducted sessions in the presence of the boy's mother, his father and both parents together, or the boy alone, and he realized by observing the parent–child interactions that the parents never sent any messages back to the child: there was never any feedback. One might say that there was no recognition of the boy's experience at any level whatsoever – not even as a wink or a word of approval or disapproval: nothing. Of course we could say, as a minimal interpretation, that the child was playing up to try to get something. While the therapist was talking with the parents and the boy was wandering around the room, tending to fiddle with everything and cause mischief, the therapist had a creative idea: he grabbed his guitar and, while continuing to talk to the parents, he played along to what the boy was doing. By doing so, he echoed the boy; it was a way of saying, "I see what you're doing; it makes sense and it's what I'm looking at". This took place on the non-verbal, implicit level and little by little the boy reacted to the therapist's music; it turned into a sort of dance between the two of them, but all the while the therapist continued talking with the parents. Was it an act of construction or deconstruction? Both at the same time.

3. Deconstruction *of* Therapy

It can be interesting to watch what we do, and the question of whether subjecting psychotherapeutic models to an evaluation is necessary or relevant has been raised in the past. The mere mention of "evaluation" is enough to cause some of us to run off screaming, and this evaluation work can also be seen as a deconstruction of our therapeutic systems, a deconstruction of therapy, a deconstruction of our position, a questioning of the role and function we have in society, and even of the political significance of the therapeutic act. Who are we? It is sometimes said that psychotherapists have replaced priests, but we prefer to argue that we don't do the same thing. Nevertheless, in terms of our role in society and our regulatory function, aren't there some similarities between us? What does it mean when such a function or profession is allowed to emerge, and what impact does it have on a society? Some models are clearly made to facilitate adaptation, submission and adjustment to social norms. Remember that Goodman used to say that if psychotherapy is about adapting or adjusting individuals to a sick society, what does it mean to conduct therapy? This idea, combined with a critique of the adjustment or adaptation function attributed to the psychotherapies of his time, is also what led Goodman to express that while one could accept a minimum level of agreement on the need for adaptation and adjustment in therapy, it was nevertheless necessary to add the term "creative". As a result, we now talk about "creative adjustment". In this context, the word "creative" should be understood in its active sense, as referring to the fact that something is created through the adjustment, not merely a poetic feature that we attribute to it for ethical reasons (since it's possible to *be* creative and *create* nothing!). When we say the adjustment must be "creative", we mean it must engage in transformation. The (active) creative act is a transformative act. While the (passive) creative act can be full of good intentions, the (active) creative act must leave a trace. I am transformed through adaptation: I adapt to the situation's conditions; when I want to sit in a chair, I adapt my body to the shape of the chair: I am transformed. Through the creative act, however, I also transform the world, creative *and* transformed in the middle voice.

Reflecting on the deconstruction *of* therapy also means reflecting on a number of concepts that are conveyed by therapy, for example. How can some concepts be iatrogenic or toxic, or have perverse effects on society? Concepts such as projection, for example, which has been seized upon by the general public, are tools available to everyone who wishes to cut off contact: "That's *your* projection!" It lets me avoid having to consider how I may or may not be responsible for something. This isn't the only example of an adverse effect of therapy: egotism, which was often denounced by Isadore From, may be another one. This culture of narcissism, reflected in Perls' prayer ("You are you and I am I, I do my thing and you do your thing, If by chance we find each other, it's beautiful. If not, it can't be helped") can also be seen as adverse effects of therapy. We might argue that it shows that this therapy probably isn't yet complete . . . but then again, how many therapies have made it to completion?

How will we, as psychotherapists, take part in constructing a context in which change becomes possible – especially a context in which choices become possible again? We shouldn't delude ourselves about the issue of choice and freedom, either. We don't have that much freedom, even in a democracy; we have a few extremely limited free spaces, and our freedom is restricted by our family background, by social conditions, by laws, by "shoulds" and "should nots", by situations; at the end of the day, the degree of freedom we have is relatively small. If we can increase our margin of freedom through therapy, even by just 1%, that's not so bad: it can make a big difference! Does freedom mean "doing what we want" or "wanting what we do"? Couldn't we connect the issue of freedom to that of engagement?

I wanted to include a reflection on several concepts that seem to corrupt not only social life, but also psychotherapy. In many respects, therapy has worked and continues to work according to a medical model. Under this model, which I refer to here in outrageously simple terms, we make a diagnosis (1st phase) and proceed with treatment (2nd phase); these are the modalities with which we evaluate the other in order to look for the most appropriate therapeutic forms. This is what is also known as the "clinical model" or "psychopathological model".

I would argue that the psychotherapeutic model must distance itself from the clinical model, that we should partially separate the traditional clinical approach from the psychotherapeutic approach, and that certain concepts, which prove fully operational in "explaining" the subject, can be toxic concepts for therapeutic support. I recently mentioned the concept of regression in a short article for *Gestalt* journal. While this concept may appear quite interesting for understanding a subject and conducting psychopathology, it often seems like a toxic concept to use in guiding a patient on a therapeutic level. I could mention many other concepts like this, such as repetition or polarities. Deconstructing therapy is also about trying to separate it from these models inspired by the medical paradigm.

4. Constructing

If we agree to leave the medical model behind, what sort of reference can we use to address construction? Following Paul Goodman and the theories suggested in *Gestalt Therapy*, I believe we can root our approach in the aesthetic model, since it is based on creating forms and giving form and structure to experience. We can draw on an aesthetic model.

What does this involve?

That will be the subject of further development in the future, particularly through the convention we are planning on this topic for 2006 (see Chapter 12 in this volume). However, we can already ask several questions: What are the qualities of forms? How can we ensure that our ethics is actually an aesthetic?

In contrast to some of the things I've said and written over the past few years, I would say something a little bit differently now – and this may be what has helped me better understand my reluctance to enter into the hermeneutical approach. I would argue that in therapeutic work, what we basically have to destroy or deconstruct are meanings and representations. The hermeneutic approach seeks to construct meaning, and we often describe therapy as the construction of meaning. Today I would go much further: *deconstruct meaning, but construct experience*. We should destroy meanings that are fixed (meaning is always relatively fixed, even if only when we elaborate it, but we tend to keep it) and construct experience. Experience must be able to function as a reservoir for the creation of meaning, since meaning should always be up for revision. I've often quoted a sentence that I came across during my psychology studies and which has stayed with me since then; Piaget, speaking to educators, said, in essence, "When you're in contact with children, don't rush to assign meaning to their experience, because for every one meaning you suggest, you shut out ninety-nine other possible meanings". In therapy, how can we work in such a way that the experience as such is what we try to build together – knowing, of course, that *his* or *her* experience will not be the same as mine in any way, and accepting that there is no common experience? How can we ensure that the other person isn't clinging to a stock of immobilized meanings, and instead that the experience can serve as a base that we can draw upon to construct and deconstruct ephemeral meanings over and over again?

> **Context:** *Within my explorations of "form", during the Summer Intensive Seminar of Institut Français de Gestalt-thérapie in 2004 on the theme "Construction/destruction of gestalts", I indulged in this little fantasy about "struction", that strange word that only has a right to exist when a prefix is attached to it. It was published in 2005, in* Cahiers de Gestalt-thérapie *no. 18.*

Chapter 15

The Language of Experience

When the question arises of how to classify gestalt therapy among the different psychotherapies that are presented to the public, several options are possible. Among them, the most frequent are humanist psychotherapies, existential psychotherapies or, more rarely, experiential psychotherapies. I prefer "experiential psychotherapy", since it refers to a concept at the heart of the gestalt formulation: that of experience, even if this concept has not given way to any profound theoretical developments, as much on the part of our founders as of their successors. In the fifties and sixties, it made sense to bring together the Third Force that distinguished itself from psychoanalysis and behaviourism under the banner of humanism. This distinction was made by reintroducing certain philosophical and ethical values to the foundations of psychotherapy. At the same time, this philosophy represented one of the last avatars of individualism, a school of thought that had marked the course of the 20th century. Without denying what could have been a major step in the development of psychotherapies and set the stage for the development of gestalt therapy, the contemporary placement of gestalt therapy in a field paradigm contains and surpasses the humanist perspective, and the reference to experience – since experience occurs at the boundary between the organism and its environment – seems more appropriate to me in the current context for considering this development.

"Experience" is the first word of gestalt therapy's founding text:

> Experience occurs at the boundary between the organism and its environment [. . .]. Experience is the function of this boundary, and psychologically what is real are the "whole" configurations of this functioning, some meaning being achieved, some action completed. The wholes of experience do not include 'everything,' but they are definite unified structures [. . .]
>
> (Perls, Hefferline and Goodman, 1951/1994, I, 1)

In these opening lines, Perls et al. position experience based on three parameters: the overall configurations of the behaviour of the contact-boundary, the construction of meaning, and the implementation and achievement of an action. Throughout the pages that follow, the authors develop their definition of other

DOI: 10.4324/9781003515760-18

constituents, but we should note that the essence of their approach to experience focuses on current experience – what is being lived – and they devote very little time to discussing experience that has been acquired, accumulated and integrated. Our language does of course use this same word to refer to what is lived in the present (*to experience something*) and what was lived and integrated in the past (*to have an experience, to have experience*). In some languages, the word for "experience" has even more meanings, such as in French, where *faire une expérience* means "to carry out an experiment"; in English as well, both "experiment" and "experience" come from the same etymological family. Experimenting thus means "trying or testing something", whereas "experiencing something" – while we may infer that something new is encountered – does not necessarily involve a deliberate, technical, rational approach, or one that is subject to protocols.

The concept's many possible uses thus present a problem that a number of philosophers have striven to articulate. This brief study does not intend to revisit the concept of experience and rival the treatments already given to it by Aristotle, Kant or the American pragmatists, nor even to restrict me to its meaning in the realm of Gestalt therapy, but only to sketch out several paths with the aim of combining these possible meanings and especially of linking language and experience in the domain of psychotherapy, since "speech easily mirrors any and all experience" (Perls, Hefferline and Goodman, 1951/1994, 7, 3).

1. And the Flesh Became Word

"The primary site of psychological experience, where psychotherapeutic theory and practice are to direct their attention, is the contact itself, the place where the self and environment stage their meetings and become involved with each other" (From and Miller, 1994).

For the gestalt therapist, contact is "the simplest and first reality" (Perls, Hefferline and Goodman, 1951/1994, I, 1), located at the boundary, and experience is the behaviour of this boundary. Contact involves "the cooperation of sense and movement (and also feeling)" (Perls, Hefferline and Goodman, 1951/1994, I, 1). The examples that illustrate this idea throughout the pages of *Gestalt Therapy*, whether expressed as nouns (appetite and disgust, approach and avoidance, sensation, feeling, manipulation, judgement, communication, struggle, annihilation, destruction, initiative and anger, etc.) or as verbs (finding food and eating it, loving and making love, attacking, entering into conflict, communicating, perceiving, learning, etc.), are always actions. Moreover, we may draw parallels between this observation and the way in which phenomenological tradition strives to transform the nouns into verbs to better highlight their active, process-related nature: contacting, thinking, saying, etc.

The practice of Gestalt therapy, which insists on centring on the process, stems much more from a verb culture than from a noun culture: "a culture of the act more than of the entity" (Robine, 2001, p. 96). On many occasions, during training sessions or conferences, I have had participants split up into groups of two or three and try having one person in each group briefly tell the others about a film or a novel, or relate a story – whatever comes to mind. An observer writes down the verbs used and their order, or at least the actions described, isolated from any anecdotal or material content. The observer then gives this list to the speaker, who is asked to think about whether this sequence of actions corresponds to something from his or her own experience in the now of the situation. Not only did the anecdote's presentation always prove to contain a description of the narrator's immediate experience, but most of the time the narrators discovered, often to their astonishment, how much their description, reduced to a process, actually had an addressee: the partner in the narrator's immediate experience. The narrators discovered that they had shared their feelings, incomplete situations, desire for encounter or avoidance, etc. with their partners. "These contacts are the structured experience of the actual present situation" (Perls, Hefferline and Goodman, 1951/1994, 9, 9). Immediate experience is expressed through verbs: the flesh is verbalized, literally becoming word. The implicitness of contact becomes explicit through the verbs used.

In therapy sessions, every narration of events or past experiences may be considered a retelling of contacts, and the succession of verbs in sequences reveals a process that, in its breadth, may say just as much about the past as about the present, or even expectations for the future. The recounting of a dream, as Isadore From demonstrated, is considered "an unaware attempt to undo a retroflected message for and to the therapist" (From, 1978), and as we know, retroflection is a form of inflecting contact that specifically concerns action.

Of course, the other words that make up the sentence are not ignored: they contextualize the verbs, and listening centred on verbs is in fact only the perceptual constitution of a particular figure/background relation, with the verbs as figures and the rest of the statement as background. The figure emerges from the background and is supported by it at the same time as it unites, organizes and structures the background.

"... to take the dynamic of experience not as a clue to some 'unconscious' unknown or a symptom, but as the important thing itself" (Perls, Hefferline and Goodman, 1951/1994, 2, 1).

2. For, And, Nor, But, Or, Yet, So

Having had experiences leads to the possibility of *having* experience. Here, experience is no longer defined in a situated time and place; it is the knowledge (know-how, skills, understanding) that is built up through "an initially sensitive perception of the world and which forms tradition through a cumulative process involving memory" (Gens, 2009, p. 9). This understanding of the concept thus refers to actions that are repeated, accumulated, sedimented and organized.

But Gadamer extends this traditional conception by expanding it beyond acquired experience: "A person who is called experienced has become so not only through experience, but is also open to new experience" (Gadamer 1960,

p. 361 French translation 1996). Gadamer's proposal is of utmost interest to Gestalt therapists, since this openness to the unknown, to the *next*, involves curiosity and the capacity to be amazed. For the dynamic to be able to enter in this direction, according to the terms of our theory of the self, the personality function of the self must not push to remain entrenched in experiences of conservative adjustments that would reduce the current situation – which is always new – to what is already known. The safety that acquired experience can offer may thereby prove neurotic, by constituting an obstacle to development and transformation.

Perls and Goodman defined the personality function as the "*verbal* replica of the self" (Perls, Hefferline and Goodman, 1951/1994, 10, 8) and highlighted three major components that preside over its construction: loyalties, morality and rhetorical attitudes. It is of course by referring to rhetoric that the link between lived experience and its expression as language takes on one of its main forms, although the authors do not limit rhetorical attitude to the mere use of language.

My hypothesis here is that the personality function forges the organization of facts of lived experience into a structure of meaning, at the same time as lived experience forges the personality function. The construction of an experience requires more than the simple accumulation of facts, moments, contacts and feelings. It also requires an organization, a rhetorical structure that will allow lived elements to be meaningfully connected. In my view, the way in which the elements of lived experience are put into relation with one another is just as crucial in constituting experience as these elements themselves. In other words: the process more than the content; the *how* more than the *what*.

Every therapist has experienced this while supporting clients who had been faced with similar difficult situations and had nevertheless taken them in in very different ways: for these events, these clients had constructed a reading of the sequence of facts in a specific linguistic logic, to such an extent that for some of them the experience had established itself as a trauma; for others it was merely an unfinished situation; for others it could have been assimilated, or served as a springboard; for others it had been erased from their memories, etc.

This articulation of segments of experience as a solid representation takes place partly through language, whether implicit or explicit, and more specifically through particular elements of language: conjunctions. Thus the "and", by uniting two or more elements, brings them together into a meaningful whole – or *Gestalt* – whose meaning is different from the sum of the meanings of their parts. Deleuze drew our attention to the primacy of this "and": "The *and* is not even a particular conjunction or relation; it is what supports all relations, the road of all relations . . ." (Deleuze and Parnet, 1977, p. 71 edn 1996).

But "and" is only one possibility for joining together the elements of lived experience. In addition to the coordinating conjunctions "for, and, nor, but, or, yet, so", which we all learned at school and, as their name indicates, coordinate experience, we have subordinating conjunctions that signal hierarchical relations between pieces of information. Grammar teaches us that these relations of subordination may be complementizers or circumstantial, with the latter referring to time, cause, manner, consequence, purpose, concession or condition (when, as, while, but, although, since, though, if), and a multitude of compound expressions that can describe the circumstances mentioned (given that, even though, according to whether, once, insomuch, etc.).

This invitation to focus on clauses in general and conjunctions in particular – an approach that is fully consistent with the methodology of gestalt therapy – is something we mainly owe to William James, one of the founders of the American pragmatist movement whose influence on the inception of gestalt therapy (by way of Paul Goodman) is indisputable, even though the founding authors of gestalt therapy never explicitly cite this influence. For James, perceiving relations between elements means perceiving the continuity of experience. He states that "[r]adical empiricism takes conjunctive relations at their face value, holding them to be as real as the terms united by them. The world it represents as a collection, some parts of which are conjunctively and others disjunctively related" (James, 1912, pp. 97–98 French translation 2005).

Furthermore, since we are on the topic of the language of experience, I am tempted to associate these essential movements of language that James calls "conjunction" and "disjunction" with the fundamental movements of the field in terms of indifferentiation/differentiation as well as the fundamental anxieties identified by Michael V. Miller in terms of overwhelming anxiety and separation anxiety. Here again, with different content, we find similar schemata.

However, if a privileged path to access immediate experience through its expression in words passes through focusing on the figure of verbs that describe contact and therefore action; and if the articulation of these immediate experiences, in order to organize them into a direction of meaning for the experience, may be revealed through conjunctions which demarcate narration; can we still consider that, to paraphrase Wittgenstein,[1] the limits of our language are the limits of our experience?

3. Is Non-Verbal Experience Linguistic?

Both postmodernists and structuralists would answer this question in the affirmative. However – and psychotherapists sensitive to non-verbal expression would not support the contrary position – we often have the sensation that something comes before language: something that often cannot be put into words – that remains ineffable.

"Since the acquisition of conscious quality on the part of an experience depends upon a context coming to it, it follows that the sum total of all experiences, having no context, cannot strictly be called conscious at all" (James, 1912, p. 115 French translation 2005).

The psychoanalyst Donnel B. Stern chooses to call these mental states that lack clarity and differentiation "unformulated experience". "Unformulated experience is the uninterpreted form of those raw materials of conscious, reflective experience that may eventually be assigned verbal interpretations and thereby brought into articulate form" (Stern, 2003, p. 37).

This progressive emergence of meaning springs more from the *creation* than from the *discovery* of any pre-existing truth such as Freud may have envisaged with his famous comparison of an analyst's work with that of an archaeologist who uncovers buried cities.[2] As with the aforementioned assimilated "experience", it will be necessary to increase the differentiation, articulation and hierarchical organization of elements.

Experience may remain unformulated as long as its author is not confronted with the necessity to communicate it to someone else. It is upon being said that this experience will articulate and organize itself, take on representations and receive a syntax. At this moment, it will take shape as symbols that have a similar meaning for a given social group. More precisely, the words used to verbally express the previously unformulated experience will be words produced by the field – in other words, contact and situation – before belonging to this or that speaker.

I invite the reader to carry out the following experiment: describe the *same* event (an anecdote, a film, a novel, a moment in your life, etc.) to several different individuals, and if possible record yourself describing it. You will immediately notice the differences between the different narrations, and you will probably be able to identify how these variations may say something about the current situation, the contact with each person, or the context.

In the psychotherapeutic situation, each individual's process of putting thoughts into words – therapist as well as client – is an emergence of the situation, and it is therefore the present situation (context, interpersonal relation, etc.) that creates the syntax of the experience, and this is all the more true if it is the first time the experience has been put into words. The more the therapist supports the possibility of an uncertain, stuttering, stammering speech pattern, the more he or she opens up the potential for what Merleau-Ponty called "speaking speech", i.e. speech that goes beyond "spoken speech" – that of a world of pre-formatted experience – this speech that Perls and Goodman called "verbalizing", in contrast with "poetry".

4. Conclusion: Experience or Meaning?

Experiencing (and its correlate in a laboratory situation such as a psychotherapy session: experimenting) brings together in the present moment all the consistency and breadth of the situation acquired at the same time as what is new. In a co-created situation, which is constantly moving, the novelty of the instant and of contacting that shows itself through acts may be partially expressed through the use of verbs. The experience acquired, which is often implicit and unformulated, may only take shape through the contact that is established as the relationship is built. These experiences, made up of acts and therefore of verbs, are structured in totalities (*gestalts*) that are narrated to others using various conjunctions. This is where the rhetoric of experience resides, and where the self's personality function is formed.

Context: *The concept of experience is essential in gestalt therapy, all the more so as it concerns what is lived, moment by moment, as well as what has been lived and accumulated. In this short note, I look at how what grammar calls "coordinating conjunctions" express the rhetoric by which we organize the meaning of our experience. This text appeared in the French* Gestalt *review, published by the Société Française de Gestalt, no. 39, 2011.*

Notes

1 The original quote from Wittgenstein reads as follows: «The limits of my language mean the limits of my world», in *Tractatus Logico-Philosophicus* (1918).
2 The archaeological metaphor runs throughout Freud's work and is particularly developed in *Civilization and its Discontents*. He went on to question it in one of his last works: *Constructions in analysis*, in *Findings, Ideas, Problems* (Freud, 1941).

Chapter 16

Ex-pression In-sists,
Im-pression Ex-ists

A Topic of Experience

At first glance, expression seems to present a paradox to the gestalt therapist, since this act – whose original meaning is "pressing out" (as in "to press the juice out of an orange") – has taken on the more general meaning of a passage from an interior to an exterior. This concept thus testifies to the legacy of a school of thought that separates interior from exterior, which Paul Goodman included in his list of "false dichotomies". The etymologies of "insist" and "exist", the two verbs used in the title of this study, are "stand inside" (*in-sistere*) and "stand outside" (*ex-sistere*), respectively.

"We don't know what we're about to say; we know once we've said it" used to say Merleau-Ponty (1969). Expression is therefore often associated with the exteriorization of the so-called interior universe, and the representation of a mental object, such as through artistic intermediaries. It may also represent an attempt to exteriorize an affect experienced by the subject when he or she pictures or exteriorizes this mental object. For this reason, the cathartic aspect of the expressive activity holds a key position, as a form of purgation and purification. With this in mind, the introduction of proposals of expression into the realm of psychotherapy opened up two associated directions for study: an analysis of psychic and representational content, and an emotional study that may work on blockages between representation, affect and emotional expression.

However, the concept of expression – like that of creation, which is often associated with it – is essentially thought of within an intrapsychic, individualist and – at best – communicational logic. Is it possible to consider it from a field perspective? If so, can this paradigm shift open new perspectives? Step by step, I would like to attempt this construction, since reflecting on expression involves a complex approach to the extent that different levels experience are mixed and unified:

– the person who expresses – in other words, the subject;
– what is expressed – the object, the content;
– the means through which it is expressed, the medium;
– the person to whom the subject expresses – in other words, the receiver.

DOI: 10.4324/9781003515760-19

Aren't these four levels already somewhat implicative of a field dynamic in line with the theory of gestalt therapy?

With his famous 1922 work *Artistry of the Mentally Ill*, Prinzhorn was doubtless one of the first psychiatrists or psychotherapists to shed light on this concept in his approach to the artwork of schizophrenics. For many years, his book served as a reference to a large number of artists, particularly surrealists like Max Ernst, Paul Eluard and André Breton, but it was only in 1984 that a French version was made available.

Prinzhorn links expression with *Gestaltung*, which he places at the heart of his theorization. The term *Gestaltung*, magnificently translated by Maldiney as "formation of forms", of course attracts our particular attention – we who practise gestalt therapy, which is after all the therapy of forms.

Prinzhorn considers that expressive movements "give concrete form to the psychic" at a given moment in which one is immediately involved since this allows communication to be established with others. These expressive movements may be automatic, instinctual or voluntary, but it is especially in Gestaltung, the formation of forms, and particularly in artistic Gestaltung that they may be considered in their entirety.

The expressive urge, for Prinzhorn (1922), is "an obscure instinctual drive that does not have its own form of discharge, in contrast to an urge in the strict sense of the term" (p. 68, French edn 1984). He also compares the expressive urge to eros, another "omnipresent fluid".

The expressive urge converges with the urge to play and the urge for adornment in the *Gestaltung* drive. (Note that Prinzhorn specifies: "Urges, drives, tendencies or needs – the choice of term makes little difference" (1922, p. 70, French edn. 1984.)

The tendency to put in order, the tendency to replicate and the symbolic urge also contribute to the formation of forms, particularly in sculpture. A "tension between expressive content and form" thus develops.

1. First Proposal

The expressive urge comes from an obscure instinctual drive and does not have its own form. It is therefore through its connection with Gestaltung *– the formation of forms – that it may be observed.*

As a further step, let us turn towards Dewey, one of the founders of American pragmatism and one of Paul Goodman's main intellectual inspirations. For Dewey, every experience begins with an impulsion, rather as an impulsion. The choice of the term "impulsion" strikes me as particularly interesting for a gestalt therapist, to the extent that it is the most consistent with our understanding of the id function of the self. The other terms often used – such as "need", which refers more to a biological level, and "desire" or "appetite", which are already loaded with the impact of representations emanating from the personality-function – are already less close to the essence of this experience. He defines experience as "a movement outward and forward of the whole organism", and also stated that "impulsions are the beginnings of complete experience because they proceed from need; from a hunger and demand that belongs to the organism as a whole and that can be supplied only by instituting definite relations with the environment" (Dewey, 1933, p. 58 1993 edn).

He then shows how every situation enables a meeting between the known and the unknown, which requires a recreation and thus allows the initial impulse to take shape and solidity because the old material – that which is attached to prior experiences – is "regenerated and gains a new life and soul".

However, Dewey effectively demonstrates that if these old materials are used in a habitual way, in routines, this cannot be termed an expressive act – only an activity. According to Dewey, in order for us to use the term "expression", what we call the ego-function in gestalt therapy must take place – in other words, the ability to select and move aside (identify and alienate). For example, if a man gets angry as a result of a passionate reaction, this anger does not constitute an expressive act because he does not think for a single moment of expressing himself – simply of unleashing his rage. An observer, however, may consider herself well-informed as to the state of the man, and that this man strongly *expresses* his anger, while in reality he is *impelled* by his emotion. Dewey thus distinguishes between expression as an experience for a subject and what an observer may consider an expressive act through rational interpretation. He differentiates between exteriorizing and expressing: "To discharge is to get rid of, to dismiss; to express is to stay by, to carry forward in development, to work out to completion." He considers it necessary for there to be "a shaping of the materials with the aim of giving body to excitement". Exposing oneself is not enough to be considered expression; it may only be a simple "discharge". It is probable that, without knowing it, Prinzhorn would agree with him here, since he only mentioned expression in connection with Gestaltung – the formation of forms.

Based on the first meaning of the verb "to express" – to press out the juice – Dewey insists on the necessity of an interaction with something external: the juicer or the foot that crushes the grapes.

The first condition for expression, therefore, is that there must be a complete experience based on the interaction between conditions and forces (excitement, emotions, etc.) of the organism and conditions and forces arising from the environment.

Second condition: the result expressed is in a way torn from the person who produced it by the pressure of these objective forces of the environment, and as a result what is produced is not untouched by these external forces.

Third condition: expression is constructed over time, not produced instantly; when complete, it has undergone a shaping and ordering that it lacked at the outset.

Lastly, fourth condition: excitement "reactivates a number of attitudes and meanings accumulated during prior experiences", which are then transformed.

As a result, when I cry out in amazement or burst into tears of joy or sadness when faced with an emotional event, this is not an expressive act, except for an observer. Based on this specific theorization, we may say that the entire self will find itself engaged in the expressive act: the impulse is triggered by the id-function of the situation, the personality-function attributes it with layers linked to prior experiences, and the ego-function provides the interface with the forces and conditions of the environment, selecting, moving aside and giving form.

2. Second Proposal

Expression implies a complete experience produced and shaped by the pressure of conditions and forces of the organism as well as conditions and forces of the environment.

Many authors agree that a large part of expression remains unconscious and therefore refer to the Freudian concept of the unconscious to approach the expressive act as well as its contents.

In 1900, Freud's discovery of the unconscious led him to write in *The Interpretation of Dreams*: "What role is now left, in our representation of things, to the phenomenon of consciousness, once so all-powerful and overshadowing all else? None other than that of a sense-organ for the perception of psychic qualities."

In gestalt therapy, referring to the hypothesis of the unconscious is optional – the unconscious is optional. Certainly, we know that entire parts of our experience are not conscious, and therefore unconscious, and we can fully accept the use of "unconscious" as an adjective, but with regard to our approach and our method, it still does not seem necessary to nominalize it: this possibility remains optional according to the relevance and consistency that we wish to attribute to it.

The first word of our founding text, *Gestalt Therapy*, is the word "experience": "Experience occurs at the boundary between the organism and its environment." Indeed, this human experience is at the heart of the understanding of psychotherapy that gestalt therapy offers, so much so that I have insisted on many occasions that gestalt therapy should be classified not among existential or humanistic therapies but among experiential therapies.

The great phenomenological psychiatrist Erwin Straus (1891–1975), in response to this assertion made by Freud, wrote:

> The truth is that experience is still "all-powerful and overshadowing all else" as it has always been; it will remain so as long as men and animals exist as individual organisms. To reach an understanding of expressive motions, one has to be careful not to confuse experience with consciousness and to see to it that a mind, a nervous system, or an id does not take the place of the living, experiencing being.
>
> (1966, p. 234)

But this concept of experience, although it has been extensively explored by philosophers, has been neglected by the majority of those in the realm of psychology and by gestalt therapists in particular, who overzealously categorized it as an obvious fact – one of these words we use without bothering to define them, along the same lines as "relation", "situation", "contact" – even "field" for a long time – and the list goes on.

It is therefore by linking expression with experience and, of course, the formation of forms that I plan to orient my remarks.

It is our experience that expresses itself and takes shape. Our experience provides structure and pre-exists any consciousness we may have of it.

3.   Third Proposal

It is experience – not the unconscious – that expresses itself and takes shape. Our experience provides structure and pre-exists any consciousness we may have of it.

Let us return to Freud's theory of the unconscious (a theory that became a postulate for many of his successors). The unconscious, need we remind ourselves, is composed of repressed content that are refused access to consciousness through the action of repression. The goal of treatment is thus to gain access to this material to allow it to be analysed. Naturally, language becomes the equivalent of consciousness and allows consciousness to be instated. Furthermore, if as Lacan (1975) stated "the unconscious is structured like a language", it becomes especially obvious that its expression by being put into words is favoured, to the extent that it would be more phenomenologically appropriate to say that, since we can only access it through language (and how can we observe it if it does not manifest itself?), the unconscious is structured *by* language.

We can easily recognize that vast swathes of our experience take place ahead of language, even if language helps give shape to our sensations. Contact with a work of art is a perfect illustration: the experience we have when faced with a painting by Goya, Cézanne or Alechinsky cannot be compared to a verbal description of the work, no matter how precise. The emotion felt when listening to Brahms' *Requiem*, a Schubert quintet, or a piece by Miles Davis or Xenakis cannot be experienced through narration.

The psychotherapist knows that many experiences arise not only from moments of the past sometimes described as archaic and from experiences that predate the acquisition of language, but also that other experiences are known but not thought about, to the extent that the discoveries and realizations enabled through psychotherapy are frequently met with "I knew it all along!", emphasizing how much the person refers to his experience first, before referring to his thought or representations.

I therefore prefer the concept of experience to that of the unconscious, knowing that part of this experience may be unformulated, to borrow the term of American psychoanalyst Donnel B. Stern.

He wrote that "Unformulated experience is the source of what experience can *become*" (2003, p. 3), and "The meanings that can be validly created from any unformulated experience are a joint outcome of pre-existing structural meanings and the emergent influence of the present moment" (2003, p. 2).

Expression therefore designates this movement that allows experience to take shape: it may take shape especially through speech, the living body, creation in general and works of art in particular. I would even add through perception of things and situations.

It also designates "everything which, being formed and determined in one way or another within an individual's psyche, is objectively exteriorized for others using one or another code of exterior signs" (Bakhtin, 1929, p. 121).

4. Fourth Proposal

Unformulated experience may take shape through verbal expression, which lets it be articulated, *or through non-verbal expression, which transforms it into* realization.

What are the conditions for making this possible?

In a recent article (2011), I had the opportunity to connect certain aspects of experience with language. I will summarize the essential aspects:

When we use the term "experience", we may refer to two essential uses, concentrated in the formulations "to experience" and "to have experience". The first refers to an immediate experience, a situation – often new – that engages me in both my initiative and my responsiveness and ability to adjust. The second refers to the sedimentation – represented or not, formulated or unformulated – of the first type of experiences and thus to their potential availability in language, affects or action.

Within the narrow limits of my remarks, I sketched how – if experience is contact, a function of the organism/environment border – language expresses this contact essentially through the use of verbs. Contact is the movement of this boundary: action, and in our language, verbs indicate action. Focusing attention on verbs and how they are connected in a sequence provides the psychotherapist with significant markers of ongoing processes, beyond the evoked content.

Still on the language level, I also mentioned how lived experience is formulated and articulated, especially based on coordinating conjunctions. As we may recall from our school years, the mnemonic FANBOYS (for, and, nor, but, or, yet, so) helps to remember these conjunctions that hide within our sentences alongside their many cousins, the subordinating conjunctions, such as "when", "because", "although", "as", "if" and a number of others. Through these conjunctions (as well as the disjunctions that they allow), we can articulate our experience and build a direction of meaning for it. Montaigne referred to these modes of articulation using a delightful expression: "verbal seams".

Of course, I do not intend to limit the passage between experience and its linguistic expression to these few aspects, but wish to address an additional dimension, since not all unformulated experience is intended for verbalization: as I mentioned, its verbal expression enables *articulation*, while its non-verbal expression enables *realization*.

Merleau-Ponty expressed this in his own way starting in his very first works: "No one will doubt that (in artistic expression) the expressive operation carries out or *produces the meaning* and does not limit itself to *translating* it. In spite of appearances, it is no different from the expression of thoughts through speech" (1945, p. 213, emphasis my own).

At the end of his life, however, he went even further, completely removing expression from the category of subjectivity.

For a long time, expression was probably thought of as a *translation* – an *exteriorization* of psychic contents. However, another approach seems possible and relevant. A philosopher whose name I've forgotten once said, "If I want to know what I'm thinking, I have to speak to someone", and I believe this principle may be expanded:

5. Fifth Proposal

Expression may be thought of not as exteriorization but as the formation of thought, speech, emotion and action. Language, emotion and action help build representations, and expression *thus forms an inseparable pair with* impression.

However, if we want to consider expression within a non-individualist field perspective as a single "drive to speak", we are led to change perspective and approach it as a social act. In this way, the expressive act should be considered particularly as the product of interaction and, more generally, the product of the social situation in which it takes place, since intersubjectivity precedes subjectivity, even when the expressive act takes place in the privacy of an office or a workshop. This is true to such an extent that the Russian philosopher and linguist Mikhail Bakhtin corrected Groddeck's famous expression "in the depths of man: id" to "in the depths of man: the other".

In the writings of Bakhtin, as in those of more contemporary writers who place intersubjectivity and field perspective as a foundation for their analyses, the expressive act can never be understood outside its relation with the concrete situation.

When Prinzhorn (1922), discussing *Gestaltung* (the formation of forms), says, "We seek the meaning of each form formed in the act of formation itself", we should not forget that this formative act is a *situated* activity.

The act of expression should therefore be understood not only as a potential meaning but furthermore as the manifestation of the situation in which it is created.

Todorov (1981, p. 148) cites several phrases from a revision project on the book on Dostoyevsky that Bakhtin was writing in the late 1950s:

> I only become conscious of myself – I only become myself – by revealing myself to others, through others and with the help of others. The most important acts that constitute self-awareness are determined by one's relation to another consciousness (to a "you"). [. . .] Every interior experience proves to be situated at the border, upon meeting another, and its entire essence resides in this intense encounter. [. . .] Man has no sovereign interior territory – he is entirely and always on a border; by looking into himself, he looks *into the eyes of another* or *through the eyes of another.*

"Situation" is what I call the overall perception of elements of the field of all the actors involved – a perception that structures the context of their encounter, gives it meaning and implicitly defines the modes of their interaction. It is a space that is constructed and limited by each of the actors involved, who are all simultaneously constructed by it and by the definition they give to it. However, it is important not to lose sight of the fact that reacting to the situation means reacting to both one's own memory and one's own affectivity, since they are part of each participant's field (organism/environment).

6.   Sixth Proposal

Expression is always situated. It is the manifestation of the situation – an activity at the boundary between the self and the world.

If subjects adapt to situations through the definitions they give them, we may further consider the way in which these situations can be a necessary constituent in the structure of expression.

Let us return to certain theories developed by Bakhtin, despite the fact that he was especially focused on language. He was among those who demonstrated that all verbal communication is an exchange of utterances – in other words, all expression is dialogic, even if the other is physically absent from the situation: this imaginary receiver is present in the form that George Herbert Mead called a "generalized other".

Beyond this statement, this other – specific or generalized – plays a decisive role in expression. I have often had the opportunity to suggest an experiment that consists in inviting someone to tell an anecdote or describe something (a film, a novel, a news item or a moment from their life) to a series of different listeners. Each time, what the speaker said was slightly different, and the differences reflected the listener's perception, the relation that existed between the speaker and each listener, and the variations of the situation. In other words, the receiver of the expression – as passive as he or she may seem – contributes to the formation of the form of this expression.

"No experience exists outside its incarnation as signs [. . .] It is not experience that organizes expression – on the contrary, expression organizes experience, gives it a form for the first time and determines its direction" (Bakhtin, 1929, p. 101 French translation 1977).

As I mentioned above, if I want to know what I am thinking, I must express myself – speak to someone. Deleuze (1969a) firmly maintained that "the other is not a structure among others in the field of perception [. . .]. He is the structure that conditions the whole field". This brings us to our next proposal.

7.   Seventh Proposal

Expression organizes experience, giving it shape and meaning. Formulated or acted – that is to say, expressed in words or in acts – experience is constructed within a given situation; the characteristics of contact, such as the reception of the expression and even its rough outline, contribute to shaping it.

Every expressive act, speech, action or work takes its meaning from what the other understands from it. It is not the intention of the person who expresses something who creates the meaning, but rather what follows the act of expression – the "next" dear to Goodman. I had the opportunity to illustrate this idea with the help of a Taoist short story which illustrates how future gives meaning to present (Robine, 2004, p. 243). It can also be illustrated through history: the Tunisian street vendor who self-immolated could have remained a news item like so many others like it, but thanks to what followed this event, it became the historic point of departure for the Arab Spring and the toppling of dictatorships. The painter who presents a new work of art surely does not offer it to the public view *with the aim of* revolutionizing painting, but the view of others gives it a meaning that may establish it as an essential turning point . . . or relegate it to the garbage heap of history – sometimes only temporarily, until another viewer assigns it another function and another meaning.

This is of paramount importance in the psychotherapeutic context, since it is I, the therapist, who will give meaning to my client's expression, but it is also my client who will give meaning to my expression, beyond my deliberate intention. For example, we all know that the tears of certain patients can move us and thereby lead us to certain types of intervention, while others can leave us unmoved, or even annoy us, and thereby lead us to other modes of presence.

8.   Eighth Proposal

The meaning of someone's expression is what the other understands it to be.

Emotion is not an "interior" experience that, at a given moment, exteriorizes itself or doesn't. What is experienced on the organism side are sensations, and when these sensations are expressed in a form, they can become emotion. "Sensings" can also become thoughts, works or actions, of course, but it is true that emotion and its derivatives, feelings, are the expression of and the most direct form taken by affects.

Alain Eraly, a Belgian social sciences researcher, takes the example of the expression of pain. When I express my pain to the people around me, my expression takes on forms that are different to those that will be created when I present them to my doctor: the situation, my desire and my expectations create a different experience, even though the pain is the same. The other is the very condition of the emergence of the self, and we have had the chance to evoke how the other and the interaction contribute to the formation of forms.

9.   Ninth Proposal

Expressing does not mean representing an interior state but rather qualifying a relation to the other.

In conclusion, let us return to the question of the body. The body is "a primary process of signification in which the thing expressed does not exist apart from the expression" (Merleau-Ponty, 1945, p. 193). Unformulated experience is one of the sources of what will become current experience. Above, we mentioned how a part of experience takes on verbal form, allowing it to be articulated, and another part assumes a non-verbal form (as action, bodily expression, etc.), allowing it to be carried out. This expression, whether verbal or non-verbal, arises from the process of collaborative construction of the field of each partner involved in the interaction, the other's main function being to define the contours and the limits of the pre-reflexive experience that we are able to create in the situation. Awareness, action, interaction and expression converge and become one.

My title linked the concepts of expression and impression, as well as those of "insisting" and "existing" – "standing inside" and "standing outside". These terms remind me of the struggle that pitted expressionist painters against the impressionists who had preceded them. The expressionists of the early 20th century – like those today we call neo-expressionists – favoured the manifestation of their subjectivity by approaching reality through its emotional component, while the impressionists wanted to describe physical reality through fleeting impressions in their contact, mainly with nature. The question remains: can there be expression without impressions?

Form cannot be taken without a link to expressiveness. Expression is a concept that resembles a rhizome, sending out its ramifications in many different directions. Its use in the psychotherapeutic context requires us to base our approach on field perspective: lack of differentiation, otherness, intentionality, perception, subjectivity and intersubjectivity, situation, spontaneity and creativity, unformulated experience, experience put into words and experience put into bodily action.

10.   Tenth Proposal

Presence is expression, manifestation. "A manifestation of energy by a person [. . .] that must be defined in terms of the whole field" (K. Lewin, quoted by English and English, 1958).

> ***Context:*** *Since the concept of expression has been with me for many years, to the point of having helped me discover gestalt therapy, it regularly comes back to haunt me and demand to be rethought from a field perspective. And how could the dialectic between "in-" and "ex-" not constantly challenge the practice and theorization of psychotherapy? What about the psyche? Is it "in" or "ex" . . .?*
>
> *This essay appeared in* Cahiers de Gestalt-thérapie *no. 32, 2014*

Chapter 17

Psychotherapy as a Situation and Contacting as Its Aesthetic Focus

Understanding an Other is most generally considered as understanding his/her psyche. And roughly speaking, psyche is defined as a by-product of one's own history. Most psychological and psychotherapeutic theories are grounded on such assumptions, and at some point these assumptions became so obvious that they stopped being considered assumptions and turned into postulates.

In the late forties and early fifties, gestalt therapy offered some seeds for a different paradigm, but looking backwards, we can observe that the radical shift suggested by this seminal work did not happen 60 years ago but more recently – let's say 20 years ago – and is still far from being widespread.

But nevertheless this paradigmatic change should have been obvious: what is called psyche is nothing but a sedimentation of ongoing contacts with human beings and with the world, and what is called history is an ongoing sequence of situations and its further organization into a narrative. That's why this revolution, in theory and in practice as well, is based on a paradigmatic shift: from individualistic – or intrapsychic – to field perspective.

I'd like to introduce some of its consequences and open some paths to further developments.

From Field to Situation

Gestalt therapy stakes its claims as belonging to field epistemology. And not just any kind of "field": the organism/environment field. This means that "field" does not exist as such, as an object that could be observed but is phenomenologically experienced by a given "organism". This field is the "lived space" (Lewin, 1936) of perceptions and actions, of feelings and meanings of any specific individual. On several occasions, Perls and Goodman, authors of our original theory, introduce the distinction between "in the field" and "of the field". Referring to "subject", "organism", "contact" as events *of* the field and not *in* the field makes it clearer, that the former phrase keeps these elements in flux, while the latter leads to a reification.

If we accept this assumption – that field is an experience and not a "thing" – it means that it appears as a "field of forces" in the here and now of every situation.

DOI: 10.4324/9781003515760-20

The therapeutic setting, whatever else it could be, is first of all a certain kind of situation. I was very puzzled years ago when I first paid close attention to a little phrase by Perls and Goodman that I had never noticed before, in which they refer to the id: "The id of the situation", they write, without any further details! (Again, it is the id *of* the situation, not the id *in* a situation!) My way of understanding this short phrase is that before it is experienced through drives, urges, needs and intentionalities, the id-function of the self arises from the situation, to be then experienced through bodily sensations which will be shaped into meanings. The situation organizes the intentionality of every agent.

This concept of situation is so commonplace that it seldom attracts attention. It is a kind of given ground, implicit and rarely focused on as a figure. However, for several dozen years, certain researchers, particularly from the Chicago School of Erving Goffman (Goffman, 1964), have placed this concept of situation at the very centre of their work. It is indisputable, however, that interest in this approach can be found earlier, in the work of John Dewey for instance.

In my first paper on situation (Robine, 2001), I provided the following illustration:

When a patient sits in front of me and tells me that he is anxious, I can choose to listen to his words not only as words in a certain situation, but also as words of the situation, as if these words were belonging to an undifferentiated field which has to be explored, instead of to an individual, the one who tells them. The individualist classical position would focus, as I used to do during many years, upon the patient's anxiety: how does he feels it, where does it comes from, what does it remind him of, which projections organize it, etc. From this position, the therapist comes to consider that he gets a more and more definite knowledge of his patient. If it may look like "natural" because it is so "usual", this position is only an unaware "choice", based on a prejudice.

Another choice, tied up with another prejudice, is to look at this anxiety as belonging first to the situation. May be this anxiety is his response to seeing me? Maybe am I making him anxious? Maybe I am making him anxious as a reaction to my seeing him? or to our meeting? Maybe "his" anxiety is actually mine? Or may it only be the atmosphere which is being created between us?

Choosing the situation as a starting point means choosing the ground as the origin of this present experience which will become figural. What I use to consider "myself" might be then considered a premature differentiation of the field. "Experience is prior to the 'organism' and the 'environment', which are abstractions from experience." (Goodman, 1972). This so-called anxiety – see above – thus refers to the knowledge the patient has about himself, i.e. what we call the *personality-function of the self,* in other words "who I think I am", and it would be more correct to say "Who I was" than "who I am" at this present moment, since the so-called "who I was" refers to previous situations while "who I am" must refer to my being in the unknown of the here and now.

How may I define a "situation"?

What I call "situation" is a whole made up of worldly, social and psychological circumstances, in which various protagonists are involved. An immediate perception of these elements from their field structures the context of their encounter, gives it meaning, and implicitly defines the modalities of their interaction. It is a specific time-space that is constructed and limited by every agent each of whom are simultaneously are constructed by it and by the definition they give to it.

And when I say that "psychological circumstances" as well as worldly and social circumstances contribute to the construction of a situation, I mean that reacting to the situation also means reacting to one's own memory and to one's own affectivity since they are part of the present organism/environment field of each agent.

In other words: *we simultaneously create and are created by the situation.*

If, as Dewey put it, "the situation controls experience" (Dewey, [1938] 1993), we therapists must be very sensitive to the different parameters that make up the situation. If Man is produced by the situations he goes through, it is important to create the types of situations that could create him as a Man. If Man is produced by his situations, he wants the power to create situations worthy of his desire. One of the goals of psychotherapy is to give – or give back – a poetic texture to life, acting upon its determining factors.

What Happens in a Situation?

Any situation is made of and creates contact. "Contact" is without a doubt the fundamental concept of gestalt therapy. Nowadays most therapies insist on their relational identity, but contact is essential prior to relationship: "Contact [. . .] is the simplest and first reality" (Perls, Hefferline & Goodman, 1951). Contact does not imply mutuality the way relationship does. To ensure that the concept of contact is used in a coherent manner, it would be preferable to systematically clarify the term "contact" by adding not only "with whom or with what" but "through which modalities" to it (Robine, 2010).

Regarding the question "With whom or what?", let us return to the introduction of Perls, Hefferline and Goodman's book: "The crucial question is: with what is one in contact? The spectator of a modern painting may believe that he is in contact with the picture while he is actually in contact with the art critic of his favorite journal." And when one focuses on transference issues, this question is of course at work.

Touching, seeing, hearing, etc. are regular modes of contact, but so are remembering, fantasizing, thinking, being excited, singing, writing, dreaming, being moved and so on. I can contact a friend by looking at him, hearing him, telephoning him, touching him, going to see him, remembering him, anticipating him, imagining him . . .

We can use the principle of noetic-noematic variations as elaborated by Husserl regarding consciousness as a basis to apply to contact. When I establish contact with someone, such as a patient, I contact this person and this person contacts me. We do not have the same contact "object", the same contents or even the same objective. (This is the noematic aspect of experience: the Other as *noema*.)

Thinking, loving, hating, imagining, etc. are acts of contact. Walking, breathing, feeling, thinking, hearing, going toward, fantasizing, dreaming, etc. are contacting types or modalities (*noesis*). With the same "object" (the "other", for example), I can have different types of contact: touching, hearing, looking, remembering him/her, feeling, projecting, cautioning, thinking of him/her, loving him/her, etc. (Robine, 2010).

Phenomenologically speaking, I can be in contact with you without you being in contact with me. For instance, from my window on the 3rd floor I can have a visual contact with you walking in the street below even though you may not have any contact with me.

Thus I might describe the way I contact you and the way I feel contacted by you, just as you might describe the way you contact me and the way you feel contacted by me, but none of us is able to describe "our" contact.

Gestalt therapy then focuses on ongoing contact modalities in the here and now of the situation, and on what I use to call "inflections" of contact (instead of "inter-ruptions of contact"), borrowing this term from Binswanger and linguistics (Rob-ine, 1997a), because we believe that "the ongoingness of the process will not be lost" (PHG, 1951).

If "contact is the first experience" (PHG, 1951), contacting an Other is a more complex operation than contacting an object or the rest of world. However, before looking at some specific aspects of contact with an Other, I would like to use one of my favourite examples to illustrate this basic feature of contact.

A client is sitting in an armchair in front of me and she levels a lot of reproaches at me, saying that I do not give her enough support. When I look at her, I can see that she is sitting on the very edge of her seat, not fully using it, using neither the back nor the arms of her chair to support her body, standing on her tiptoes on the floor. Through this body language, she shows me that she does not use the available support from her environment. We may assume that the way she contacts an Other resembles her "material" contact with the world and that some of her patterns of contacting are subjected to inflections.

Contact with an Other

Merleau-Ponty wrote: "We don't know what we are saying, we know after having said it," and I even would like to go one step further and add my own assumption: "If I want to know what I think, I have to speak with someone."

The first sentence of gestalt therapy's foundational text is "Experience occurs at the boundary between the organism and its environment" (PHG, 1951)

Dewey had shown that for any kind of expression, an interaction is necessary between some forces of the organism (excitement, emotions, etc.) and forces from the environment, and that the result is somehow pulled out by this pressure from the environment and therefore is not free from it.

It means that every expression, verbal or non-verbal, is always situated, always happens in contact. It is an outward sign of the situation, an activity of the boundary between oneself and the world. This phenomenon has a lot to do with what Ruella Frank calls "kinesthetic resonance" (Frank, 2013).

What happens in contact could be no longer considered as an exteriorization of some prior subjectivity but rather the formation of thought, speech, emotion, action, etc. Any expressive act, any contact – in both its form and its contents – are products of interaction and, broadly speaking, of the social situation. The Russian philosopher and linguist Mikhail Bakhtin in his project for a revision of his book about Dostoyevsky, wrote beautifully:

> I become aware of myself, I become myself only in self-revealing for an Other, through an Other, thanks to an Other. Most important acts, constituent of self-awareness, are determined inside a connection to another consciousness (to a "you") [. . .] Every inner experience in fact turns out to be situated at the boundary, it meets an Other and its whole essence lies in this intense encounter [. . .] Man does not own any inner sovereign territory; he is completely and always on a boundary; looking inwards, he looks into an Other's eyes or through an Other's eyes.
>
> (Bakhtin, quoted by Todorov, 1981)

Even when no Other is physically present, every expression is dialogic, in contact with a "generalized Other" (Mead, 1934). Or, to use Deleuze's words, "The Other is not a structure among structures within the perceptive field [. . .] He is the structure that conditions the whole field" (Deleuze, 1969a).

Sometimes, during introductory workshops on working in a field perspective, I propose an experiment: in dyads, describe a sequence of a film or novel to a member of the group.

An experiment could be to have the participant describe the same short sequence to different people and to notice the differences in narration.

Another experiment could be to hold a kind of mini-session on "what I am telling you through this telling", phenomenologically unfolding the process included in the narrative. Participants always notice that the excerpt they have chosen from the film or novel is an unconscious means to tell the other something belonging to their contact or to their unfinished issues actualized by the situation.

Similarly the differences in narration in the first experiment can reveal some specific features of their contact in this situation.

However, let us return to Bakhtin: "There is no experience outside its incarnation into signs [. . .] It is not experience that organizes expression but, contrarily, expression that organizes experience, that for the first time gives it a form and determines its direction" (Bakhtin, 1929).

Bakhtin may have been one of the first to claim what is nowadays well known: that no word, no phrase, no sentence has any meaning until it is completed by the answer from the Other: his answer gives meaning to what I have just said. To Merleau-Ponty who wrote (see above) "We don't know what we are saying, we know after having said id", I add: ". . . we know after having said it *to an Other, and through his answer this Other gives meaning to my words.*" This, of course, is of huge importance in the therapeutic situation.

I used the topic of "expression" (verbal or non-verbal) to develop this fundamental topic of contact because it is one of the major parameters in differentiating between contact with human beings and contact with objects of the world. Expression gives form to experience. "Unformulated experience", as Donald Stern (Stern, 2003) would say, is like clay for a sculptor: it has no prior shape or form, it will be shaped and formed through contact.

Form is a major concept in our approach, not only because it is an approximate translation of "Gestalt" but also because we consider that we can only approach human experience through the forms it takes on: we cannot observe any desire or urge except through the forms they assume. Emotions are forms given to what is felt, symptoms are forms, language is form, contact does not exist without a specific form, and relationships have forms. So does the therapeutic setting, a form given to what Goffman named "working acceptance" (Goffman, 1988).

If situations shape experience, if contact takes different forms according to situations and interactions, the ongoing events of therapeutic encounter must be considered according to appropriate references, and we can easily understand that medical or scientific criteria are far from focusing on "forms". Adequate reference must be found in aesthetics.

When I refer to "aesthetics", I refer to the meaning given by Baumgarten, the concept's founder, an 18th-century German philosopher, who created the term "aesthetic", from the Greek *aisthétikos*, to refer to the science of sensory knowledge, which he contrasted with the knowledge of conceptual objects. In aesthetics, it is the senses and sensory objects that enable us to recreate both meaning and existence, and to create new forms of subjectivation.

Aesthetics must be differentiated from the philosophy of art. Of course, art is not entirely foreign to the aesthetic approach: art is one of the domains in which aesthetics can be brought into play. Art thus becomes not just a privileged form of aesthetics but nearly its most paradigmatic form. I do not claim that psychotherapy is an art, but I do consider that we may draw upon the phenomenology of artistic creation in order to define the therapeutic act. As Laura Perls puts it:

> The main concern of the artist is certainly not the "exercise of aesthetic transformation" of truth into beauty, but rather the organization of a multitude of various disparate, incompatible experiences that threaten the individual or society with disintegration – therefore are experienced as ugly – into a meaningful, integrated whole, a unity within which they make sense and which therefore is or may be experienced as beautiful.
>
> (Perls, 1992)

Kant wanted to reconcile what is felt and what is thought. There are no criteria for judging a work of art because the work *is* its own criterion. For Kant the work of art is *nomothetic*, that is, it enacts its own laws. In fact art has one characteristic that sets it apart from other human activities and institutions: while other human activities are judged according to their relative efficacy and usefulness in terms of the values they embody, work of art refuses any such reference to its usefulness, external criteria or accepted values.

Paul Goodman, one of the co-founders of gestalt therapy, positioned psychotherapy within this Kantian perspective to a certain extent when he wrote, "The fact that the Gestalt has specific observable psychological properties is of capital importance in psychotherapy for it gives *an autonomous criterion of the depth and reality of the experience*" (PHG, 1951).

The aesthetic aspect of gestalt therapy locates the origin of experience within the senses: feelings, sensations, and perceptions. As Dan Bloom wrote,

> If we understand the figure/background process as essentially one that is sensed, felt, perceived, we can then notice the fluidity or fixity of this through its aesthetic qualities. Experience may then be appreciated for its intrinsic form rather than by comparison to extrinsic content-based standards.
>
> (Bloom, 2005)

Contact – again, which Perls and Goodman define as "the first and simplest reality", (PHG, 1951) has observable properties that we grasp through our senses. The authors draw on aesthetic terminology when they describe the figure: clarity, brilliance, liveliness, meaningfulness, sharpness, intensity, unity, uniqueness, harmony, grace, fluidity, vitality, rhythm and symmetry, to mention just a few. These are terms drawn from the same semantic field that describes physical activity, consciousness, breathing, vocalizing and so on. These terms are not based on clinical, social or cultural criteria but on direct sensory experience.

> It is not necessary to have theories of "normal behaviour" or "adjustment to reality" except in order to explore. When the figure is dull, confused, graceless, lacking in energy (a "weak Gestalt"), we may be sure that there is a lack of contact, something in the environment is blocked out, some vital organic need is not being expressed. The person is not "all there", that is, his whole field cannot lend its urgency and resources to the completion of the figure.
>
> (PHG, 1951).

"Form is the place where an organism meets its environment" wrote von Weizsäcker. For Dewey, "Form is the way in which we shape and integrate our experiences". It is form that selects and intensifies the spatial and temporal aspects of perception. The need for form and the experience of development are intimately linked: development is the organizing of experience over time, and form is what renders the nature of this organization explicit.

It was above all Hans Prinzhorn who crystallized an artistic and psychiatric theory around a proposition that I have often had occasion to quote, "We seek the meaning of every form that is formed by the act of formation itself".

"The structure of a situation is the internal coherence of its form and content" (PHG, 1951), claims Goodman. It is therefore both our function and our responsibility to help define the situation in such a way that we can apply aesthetic criteria when structuring the experience.

On the subject of art and therapeutic work, French philosopher Felix Guattari posited: "What is important is to know if a work leads effectively to a *mutant production of enunciation*" (Guattari, 1992).

Context: *Invited in 2013 to make gestalt therapy better known to the philosophers, psychoanalysts, psychotherapists and theologians who gather each year in Cambridge, MA for the "Psychology and the Other" symposium, I tried to approach this introduction from unusual paths, no doubt quite different from those that have brought gestalt therapy to the general public as well as to neighbouring professions. Sheila McNamee, a major representative with K. Gergen of Social Constructionism, was the respondent. This lecture (and McNamee's response) appeared in* Cahiers de Gestalt-thérapie *no. 32, 2014.*

How Situations Create Encounters

Chapter 18

Self-Reference, Self-Disclosure, Self-Implication of the Gestalt Therapist

Therapist disclosure is an issue that has been debated by psychotherapists since the beginnings of contemporary psychotherapy. This debate is fuelled by paradoxes, scientistic arguments or beliefs, and theoretical presuppositions. Freud, for example, posited that the therapist "should be impenetrable to the patient, and like a mirror, reflect nothing but what is shown to him" (Freud, 1912). His conception of the "impenetrable" may seem somewhat paradoxical if we remember he willingly told his patients about his own dreams and childhood memories. A strange blindness still allows certain contemporary psychotherapists and psychoanalysts to believe in the silence of their silence, their benevolent neutrality, the whiteness of the projection screen they offer their patients.

The international literature on the issue of therapist disclosure generally adopts the attitude that "it depends!". The relevance of the therapist's self-disclosure depends on its content, the reasons for this disclosure, the personality of the patient to whom it is addressed, the situation and circumstances, etc. Research has shown that therapist disclosure has both positive and negative consequences for the patient's development. Reading these accounts has only confirmed my questions and uncertainties regarding the ethical recommendations and opinions that have been published, such as the research that has been done on the impact of this type of disclosure. Based on my psychotherapeutic experience as both a patient and a supervisee, and as psychotherapist, a supervisor and a trainer, I could just as easily demonstrate the advantages of these choices as I could their disadvantages, since they have both positive and negative effects.

If, as Yalom (1985) argues, "more than any other single characteristic, the nature and degree of therapist self-disclosure differentiates the various schools of psychotherapy", there should be some consistency among our theoretical choices at work in our decision or refusal to disclose. In this chapter, I intend to focus on several aspects of this connection.

1. In Whose Service?

My first question is this: who is the therapist's self-disclosure meant to serve? Although it supposedly nourishes the therapeutic process by strengthening the therapist–patient

DOI: 10.4324/9781003515760-22

bond and injecting authenticity into their relationship, it is not always clear whether this practice primarily benefits the patient. A certain narcissistic complacency on the part of the therapist in narrating his or her own experience cannot be excluded. The patient's consequent recognition of the therapist confirms this hypothesis, especially if we admit that the intentionality of an action is more likely revealed through its effects than by an explanation of the plans of the person acting.

Allaying one's own anxiety, ensuring one's knowledge through experience, providing evidence and justifications, and modelling are among the potential issues involved.

Marthe is a student in her early twenties. She comes to see me for a preliminary interview with the intention of starting psychotherapy. Throughout our interview, she talks so much that I cannot get a word in edgewise and am unable to ask her any questions or provide information on the work we might consider doing together. I make another appointment with her for a second preliminary interview and tell her that next time, we can talk about the psychotherapy itself and implement a system for our meetings, if she intends to continue.

She begins this second interview as the first, with a very dense speech flow, without any pauses but without any apparent affect, either. I worry about once again not being able to make my way into the conversation, if only to show her a "little something" of my way of working by experience, and especially in order to jointly define our working methods. The opportunity suddenly arises: her speech slows and tears come to her eyes as she talks about a painful episode from her childhood; there is a short gap in her flood of words and I decide to get my foot in the door with a trivial phrase like, "I'm touched to perceive your emotion and your attempt to hold onto it when you talk about this time in your life . . ." Her reaction is immediate and cracks like a whip: "Oh no! Never say anything like that again! I don't want to know what moves you and what doesn't. I know myself well enough to be sure that if I know I can affect you in such and such a way, I'll conform to that behaviour in order to reach you. I want to stay free!"

Clearly, I was the one who needed to say something, to make my existence known, to make room for some sensitivity in a disaffected narrative flow . . . She forcefully reminded me *who was at whose service.*

2. Twisting Figures

One of the gestalt therapist's major tasks is to let the patient build a strong, clear, assertive gestalt. With the psychotherapist's help, the patient must be able to find a common thread among scattered elements of his or her experience. This is one of the more delicate phases of the process, in which the aesthetic qualities of the therapist are applied to the form taking shape, and his or her qualities of firmness help *hold onto* the emerging theme together with the patient, without becoming complicit in siren songs, interruptions, or habitual or tempting circumventions.

The therapist actively contributes during this construction phase, sometimes using material drawn from his or her own experience to participate in the task. The difficulty therefore lies in contributing in a way that is sufficiently discreet and relevant, so that the material provided does not decentre the figure being developed. This means remaining at the service of the figure being constructed, not becoming the figure that vies for the attention of a patient who may be open to any and all loopholes available in this delicate phase of withdrawing from confluence.

My first encounter with gestalt therapy takes place in the mid-seventies. After several years of psychodrama group work, I encounter another form of group psychotherapy. What I am most sensitive to in terms of the novelty of this first experience is that it offers a form of work in which expressing one's emotions and affects is welcomed.

I'm going through a difficult phase of my life: a low-level crisis, full of retroflections and silences; questions and doubts; uncertainties, sorrows and disappointments. After a few hours, I discuss these issues with some difficulty because nothing is clear – I don't know where to start things; I don't know how to put what I experience into words; I'm floundering. After a few minutes, the gestalt therapist, with his magnificent dyed-in-the-wool English accent, tells me about his experience: "You know, Jean-Marie, I am sensitive to your experience and I know that pain. A few years ago, I also experienced a period of depression and I even tried to kill myself . . ." and continues telling me in great detail about his psychiatric hospitalization, "the intensity of his case", etc.

The moments when his words have a soothing effect on me are short-lived. At first confusedly, then more and more clearly, my anger grows: I feel robbed. He has stolen my experience, robbed me of my expression and crushed my emotion. He is more *than me: what is my humble melancholy next to his major depression? What right do I have to complain when others may be suffering from something oh-so-much more serious? And childhood memories come back to me in which my suffering went unheeded on the grounds that others were suffering for far more serious reasons; my claims that I didn't like a certain type of food were not listened to, considering the famine faced by millions of children in China who were less fortunate than me . . .*

I clumsily express that I am not interested in his story, as it does not help resolve my own. The group comes to my rescue, offering their support. The therapist looks surprised, even shocked, and he withdraws to an adjoining room. Ten minutes later he returns . . . to tell us in a voice from beyond the grave, "You don't like me, so I'm going away; I'm stopping this group and leaving you." He proceeds to do just that, to our general amazement.

This is another example where not only do the therapist's needs take precedence over those of the patient, but the therapist also inflects the figure under construction, giving it a different meaning than the one the patient is struggling to express, and thus tries to become the focus of the group's attention.

When it comes to contributing to the development of the figure, the therapist is biased in the choice of materials that he or she will choose to use and engage in the situation. Certainly, whatever they are, they will never be neutral. The therapist's involvement in the situation, coupled with his or her personal ethics and clinical experience, is among the determinant factors of his or her choices. Knowing exactly why these choices are made as they are seems just as impossible as drawing up a list of criteria that rationally explain why a painter chooses one shade of yellow rather than another for his or her next brushstroke.

3. Contact or Relationship?

In fact, the responses (in the form of action) to this question of disclosure reveal the essence of each professional's conception of psychotherapy – sometimes explicitly but more often implicitly – and the epistemology that he or she chooses to employ.

One of the more common epistemological confusions among supporters of our approach is the confusion between the concepts of "contact" and "relationship". In everyday language, the two words are often used interchangeably. Following in the footsteps of certain philosophers and phenomenologists (Sartre, Maldiney, Szondi, Colli[1] and others), the theory of gestalt therapy defines the contours of the concept of contact much more precisely. Furthermore, the original theory of gestalt therapy says nothing about the "relationship", therapeutic or otherwise; in this respect, it resembles many other psychotherapeutic approaches that only conserve one single ingredient of the "relationship" in their theories, reducing it to transfer, interaction, connection, bond, projective identification, etc. depending on the case. Contact, defined as "the simplest and first reality" (Perls, Hefferline and Goodman, 1951/1994 I, 1), designates the basic operation in which a particular organism connects with its environment. It is the immediate awareness that we have of the field and behaviour directed at it. Even if contact involves a connection between a subject and an object experienced as distinct from the subject – whether the object in question is a thing, an idea or a person, it postulates a "with" (Latin etymology: *cum-tangere*) – this term cannot be systematically replaced by the term "relationship". The way I make visual contact with a painting, a food or a landscape does not involve any reciprocity in the experience; the same cannot be said for a relationship, even though elements in a relationship are not necessarily identical or symmetrical.

The theoretical corpus of gestalt therapy provides conceptual and methodological equipment to put contacting into practice (contacting being how a subject contacts and is contacted by the world). This system cannot be used to describe the "relationship".

Of course, this contacting is deployed in a relationship, and we should keep in mind that a relationship is a therapeutic means rather than an end in itself[2].

Psychotherapist self-disclosure may prove to be a particularly relevant instrument in identifying modes of contacting, especially those of the patient contacting his or her therapist. This is what I will attempt to demonstrate, while applying the two ethical limits mentioned and illustrated above.

4. Engaged in the Situation

Gestalt Therapy, our founding text, contains a concept that I consider key to the theoretical construction of our approach, although it remained unnoticed for a long time: the "id of the situation". It is unsurprising that this concept has remained in the shadows, considering that the authors hardly gave themselves the means to further define their proposal. With this concept, they lead us once again into a field perspective, even though the "id", so central to psychoanalysis, could be seen as *the* intrapsychic concept par excellence. In the tradition of psychoanalytic thought, and to use the original French title of the book in which Groddeck introduced the concept that Freud later seized upon, *Au fond de l'homme: cela*[3] ("Deep within man: id"). The id is thus located "deep within the human being", even "deeper" than the unconscious, which is considered a secondary structure while the id is theorized as a primary structure.

Perls and Goodman later propose the concept of the "id of the situation", a radical relocation of the id: should the id be sought in the situation? The consequence I take from this proposal is that the emergence of the id is rooted in the situation, intentionality is produced by the situation, and the id is formatted in terms of desire, need and appetite through the ego function of the self, not without intervention by the personality function. The field is primary and foundational; it is driven and organized by the self, which is itself a function of the organism and what surrounds it, which in turn creates and is created by the field.

Whenever two people are in each other's presence, the situation they create and develop is a contact situation. This situation generates the emergence of an id that is specific to each of them: that is to say, a push; a direction of meaning and meanings; an intentionality in which the other has a place, no matter how small or how vehemently denied it may be.

In other words, being in another's presence creates a feeling in each person that may remain implicit and non-conscious but nevertheless spurs being-with-an-other. I would even speculate that in any situation where people are placed in each other's presence, the desire always arises to affect the other and to create a specific feeling in him or her ("Look at me!", "Recognize me", "Leave me alone – don't talk to me", "Show me that you see me", "Love me", "Want me", etc.).

When asked about his aim or how he wishes to affect the other, the subject may only provide a response shaped by his conscious intentions or deliberate plans, or rebuilt by the ego ideal, the representations he has of himself and other factors that make up what gestalt therapy calls "the personality function". However, this method leaves hardly any room for consideration of the now, the novelty of the situation, the unknown or the surprise of a modality of presence toward the other that we never imagined.

So how can I find out about the impact of my presence on the other, beyond the assumptions and representations that I have about myself? By asking the other how he or she is affected by my contact and its variations from moment to moment. "Everything takes place as if the other's intention inhabited my body, or as if my intentions inhabited his", wrote Merleau-Ponty (1945, pp. 215–216)[4] beautifully. As such, the psychotherapist's disclosure of his or her experience, strictly rooted in the here and now of the situation and its impermanence, is fully justified.

Esther is about forty years old. She is a psychotherapist and finished her train-ing as a gestalt therapist with me and my team around twelve years ago. Since the end of her training, I had not had the chance to see her or hear about her until this session, which kicks off a professional development programme that she signed up for. I offer to conduct a session with a volunteer so that we will have shared mate-rial for analysis and theoretical and methodological development. The entire ses-sion was recorded on video; the transcript below contains selected extracts. Only the patient's name has been changed.

In the first part of the session that I summarize here, she is overcome by sobbing and her words are hard to make out between the spasms of her tears.

[. . .]

E: *I've never felt loved – or appreciated – I'm sure of that! – In my life – I've always tried hard – to make them recognize me – as a girl – and never – I never got it . . . So that now – I know – and I don't look for that recognition anymore . . .*

Now, I need – my husband to recognize me . . . I guess – I chose – the spouse that I chose – it's because it's the same thing! The relationship is the same – I'm – in a relationship with him – as I was – with my mother . . . And now, what I need – is for my husband to rec-ognize me. I don't think he realizes what I'm say-ing to him! I try to tell him to recognize me . . . and he says I'm bothering him, I'm weighing on him, or I'm not mature. Why should he say anything if I do something well?

And I personally need to be told!

And if he isn't able to give me that, I don't want to stay with him anymore. It's hard for me to tell him that, even though I try, and he assaults me and cuts me off because he says I'm aggressive when I speak, because I'm afraid – I'm not sure of myself . . .

JMR: *Esther –I'm very sensitive – to – how your pain manifests itself. – More than tears – I have the*

	impression that I perceive – a form – of choking – of suffocation.
E:	*I don't know . . .*
JMR:	*How is your breathing right now?*
E:	*I don't think I'm breathing very well. It's still stuck here* (points to her diaphragm).
JMR:	*Earlier, when we started the session, you said a few words about yourself. You said that at the moment you had a lot of sadness and you cried a lot, especially when you were alone. What makes you choose to cry* preferably *when you're alone?*
E:	(Crying) *Because I feel alone. When I'm around other people, I guess I have to be an adult – you know, sensible – so crying, I keep to myself . . .*
JMR:	*And to ourselves, too!*
E:	*The urge to cry, here . . . at first I didn't want to – I made sure that it didn't happen. I thought it wasn't a good way to start with this group! And then I thought I didn't care. My tears and sadness showed up because I felt really glad to have been chosen to join this group; it showed me that people liked me; it gave me a kind of recognition.*
JMR:	*And is this the kind of recognition that you need?!*
E:	(Nods).
JMR:	*And this request for recognition – don't you seem to completely focus it on your husband?*
E (sobbing):	*Yes. I had a hard time. I started to cry a month or two ago, but I didn't know . . . I was sad, I was sad . . . I didn't understand: first I felt sad and sad and sad, and then I felt lonely. I need a relationship – I want the relationship; I need it! Period!*
	[. . .] (She continues and develops the topic)
JMR:	*So . . . in the situation we're in right now, you and me, I'm wondering if what's happening isn't something related to what's happening in your life: I perceive your suffering, I can understand it, but I can't seem to* feel *what your need may be in our situation, at this moment of* our *encounter.*
	[First step in the psychotherapist's self-disclosure as an attempt to lead the patient to a component of the experience which she does not seem to be paying attention to: the now, the presence of an other, the recipient of her expression]

E:	*I guess that coming to sit here and making the effort to explain how I feel* (starts sobbing again) *somehow forces me to make sense of what I feel.*
	I just realized that I probably needed . . . and I chose you . . . so that you'd tell me that I needed this to grow in a healthy way.
JMR:	*You expect me to confirm that your need is legitimate.*
E [nods slowly, crying]:	*Yes, that's what I need . . . And to hear that I'm not crazy . . .*
JMR:	[Silence – thinking]
	Something strange is happening . . .
	As far as I can tell, you're intensely showing me your sadness . . . And yet it produces quite a dry reaction in me, as if I weren't very sensitive to it! And I'm surprised that I'm so little affected by what you're saying.
	I'm very surprised! I'd like to understand . . . What's keeping me from being affected? I think it probably has something to do with how it's taking place.
	[Second step in the therapist's increasing use of self, since the first step does not seem to have been fully recognized by the patient]
E[Silence, calmer]:	*Maybe I'm making a mistake by asking for someone to hold my hand or recognize me . . . I've been told that I go looking for flaws or that I'm going in circles!*
JMR:	*Do you feel like the same thing could happen with me? Even though I don't want to tell you that –*
	[Third attempt, invitation to open one's eyes to the situation in the now]
E:	*No! No!*
JMR:	*So why can't I be truly affected?*
E (Shrugs):	*I don't know . . .*
JMR:	*If my feelings aren't stirred at this moment of my encounter with you, it's almost as if I don't feel like a real person . . .*
	So why wouldn't I be a real person around you? You're usually someone who affects me! I have affection for you, and you know it!
	[I take an extra step in my invitation to draw on what is happening in the here and now of her contacting. My own insistence starts to cause trouble because I am afraid of generating shame in Esther. To carefully focus her attention on the now rather than on sweeping

generalizations, I specify that my experience constitutes a figure *in the now* and – surprisingly – contradicts the usual affect that is part of the foundation of this figure]

E: *Yes, I know.*

JMR: *So how is it that in this moment, which is intense and dramatic, I have a heart of stone?*

[Additional step to insist on putting feelings into figures, with even more confrontational words, since she gave me a sign that she heard me ("Yes, I know") when I mentioned the background I remembered ("I have affection for you, and you know it")]

E: *It's occurred to me that I might be playing the victim, or the little girl . . . but I don't think I'm playing a manipulative victim.*

JMR: *No, me neither.*

E: *I don't know.*

JMR: *Something's becoming more specific, now that I'm trying to put all this into words with you. I think I see you as being all alone . . . and not at all with me.*

[Meaning is constructed little by little and illuminates what is happening. I take the risk of mentioning the hypothesis that is being created for me, since the escalation of our interaction could lead her toward a humiliating stalemate.]

E: *Yes, I am alone – I feel lonely . . .*

JMR: *Yes, but when are you alone?*

E: *All the time – my whole life . . .*

JMR: *We aren't in "your whole life". Life contains particular moments: moments of encounter, moments of isolation, moments of encounter, moments of isolation . . . Right now, we're trying to encounter each other. And yet I think I see you alone, locked up inside your pain and your solitude, as if I weren't there for you. And as a result . . . I'm not affected. As if perhaps you weren't addressing a person but a function.*

It may not be just what I'm saying: I'm with you in trying to understand what's happening. . .

E: (Thinking silently)

Let's see . . . I know I'm alone; I know I'm loved. I kind of have the feeling that the recognition I never got from my mother my whole life, the same thing is happening in my marriage, and . . . and . . . and . . . Maybe I'm asking for too much but it's something I need.

JMR: *I can offer a hypothesis, which seems incomplete to me and certainly doesn't cover everything that's happening with your husband or your mother. It's something about the "how": the "how with an other".*

I suggest that you try something now: try to reach me now – to make sure that I'm with you and that I'm affected and concerned by you . . .

[I go one step further: self-disclosure no longer seems necessary; from now on, all I need to keep contributing to the construction of the figure is my commitment]

E: (She shakes her head, shrugs and cries to say *I don't know, I don't know . . .*)

JMR: *I don't know how, either – let's try!*

Does it interest you? Are you interested in me being present in your experience? Completely present, including emotionally?

E: *I know that . . . I don't know, Jean-Marie!*
. . . Maybe it has something to do with me?
I sense that you like me . . .
I don't need your approval. I sense that you like me and I don't need your approval.
You're someone I value. Maybe here isn't the best place to talk about it but you help me understand . . . othewise I'd just be crying and crying all the time about these problems! That's why I wanted to work with you, to spot things that escape me. I've actually thought a lot more about this whole issue than what I may have said. I don't spend all my time crying like I'm doing now.
(Silence; she looks at me)
I get your smile. Thank you for your smile.
(Cries)
Could you kiss me?

JMR: *In this moment, what meaning would that have for you?*

E: (Crying) *I guess it would be the recognition that I haven't gotten!*

JMR: *I'd like to hold you in my arms, but I feel I have some reservations . . .*

E: *Me too – I'm not looking at it very clearly.*

JMR: *I could do it, but then again I imagine being . . . dry! If I were to take you in my arms, I'd prefer to do it . . . warmly! With the warmth I usually feel toward you, which has not yet been awakened.*

E: *Yes, I know; this isn't the time.*

JMR:	*Whether it's the right time or not . . . how can we create this warmth between us?*
E:	*Suddenly, an image just came to me: when I ask my husband for things, he doesn't say anything or he talks about something else, and maybe it doesn't affect him! That just sprang into my mind.*
JMR:	*I have the impression that your tears are not addressed to me . . . You aren't "sending" your tears to me. You're crying from yourself to yourself!*
E:	(Nods and cries) *Yes.*
JMR:	*So that's why it isn't about me! And maybe it's the same way with your husband? Maybe?*
E:	(Shrugs) *Maybe!*
JMR:	*How could you send me your tears?*
E:	*I don't know.*
JMR:	*You can try . . . but not by thinking!*
	(Silence)
	Can you imagine that I could receive your tears?
	(Makes hand gesture in the shape of a cup in her direction)
	How could you make sure that I receive them? (Silence)
E:	*[. . .] I need you to love me and to take me in your arms, but . . .*
	Now, I'd put myself in this position (Crying, she points to the corner of the room and gestures as if to place a ball there)
JMR:	*But that's what you know how to do* (she nods)*: use your tears to cut yourself off!*
E:	*Use my tears to cut myself off? Cut myself off from what?*
JMR:	*From the other – from contact!*
	(Silence)
	If you go into the corner, you'll cut off contact!
E:	*I think I should stop crying!* (For the first time she takes a handkerchief from behind her)
JMR:	*I have another suggestion to make, which is not to take you in my arms to give you a hug, but to lend you my shoulder for a moment – so you can cry on it.*
E:	(Nods)
	Oh, yes – I prefer your shoulder to a hug!
	(I approach her slightly; she also comes closer to me and lays her head on my shoulder, sobbing for 30 seconds. Then she pulls away)
	It is as if I had to bear all the responsibility, and by letting me cry on your shoulder, you gave me a little rest

from all that. Asking you to hold me was probably also an attempt to get some rest! That's it! Taking a break from all this responsibility . . . Yes, I can rest a little – I think that's it. I feel like I have to carry this burden all by myself.

I feel alone – that's all I've ever known.

That's always how I saw my mother: pulling her own weight with no help from anyone else, and there are a lot of times when I feel like I have to do the same.

JMR: *Yes . . . Yes . . . To such an extent that you don't notice that there are people alongside you who could help you bear the load?*

E: (Slowly nods, in silence)

Yes! I think that's where it comes from . . . (She keeps nodding) Yes . . . I think that's it . . . (Long silence)

JMR: *You say you need the other to give you some sign of recognition, but . . . for the other to be able to give you those signs, maybe you also have to make him or her exist . . . in your experience?*

E: (She nods in silence)

Yes, that's what I saw! Thank you!

JMR: *Shall we stop there?*

In this illustration, the therapist (i.e. myself) provides the patient with access to his feelings, without knowing where his expression will lead, but with the hope that once the patient knows that her expression has an impact on others, she will include this as one of the parameters of the experience. As the patient says herself, time and again in her own therapy she had the chance to explore the contents of her suffering, the impasse of her demand and the origin of her impossible expectations. Did she have the opportunity to learn something about the now, and how to better assess the impact of her mode of contacting? We can see how she remains stationary for most of the session in her usual system and how, suddenly, something opens up: she listens, and "the other" exists. What will she do with all this? When I see her again, about six months later, she tells me about her integration of this session and the radical transformation of her relation to the other that ensued. She even sends me her husband's thanks!

The psychotherapist's self-disclosure thus takes on its full meaning: the aim is not so much to reveal elements of one's personal history and experience, or even to discuss one's career and professional guidance, as is often the case, but rather to talk about oneself as an affected other – almost a "generalized other" – thereby restoring the patient as a "being-with".

One of the major difficulties of this form of self-exposure lies in the use of language. It is easy to hurt the patient, making him or her bear the responsibility for the occasionally unpleasant feelings that the therapist may experience during a session, thereby putting the patient in a position of shame. How can we disclose our boredom or anger – if it may be of some use to the situation – without hurting the patient? Rather than opening something in the current experience, such an expression on the part of the psychotherapist may be even more likely to close it off, implicitly guiding the patient toward further retroflection or complacency.

Self-disclosure on the part of the psychotherapist, it must be remembered, is not an end in itself. To me, it does not even appear to be a necessary principle. It is only one of the tools of the trade that may be used to analyse contact and its transformation: one of many possible forms of the gestalt therapist's engagement in the situation.

Context: *One of the widespread misunderstandings of the development of the field perspective in gestalt therapy has resulted in the therapist's immoderate use of self-disclosure during sessions. As if "field" meant "common field", and as if this so-called "common field" implied a symmetry and reciprocity of self-exposure, or as if Martin Buber's famous I–Thou and dialogical attitude were to manifest itself in this "posture". Invited to Brasilia and then Moscow to sketch out the contours of this questioning, I took up some of its technical and ethical aspects in the French review* Gestalt *no. 33, in 2007, before leading a number of international seminars on the subject.*

Notes

1 Sartre (1995), especially p. 400 ff; Maldiney (1990a; 1990b); Szondi (1983); Colli (1982).
2 There is much more to say about this topic, at a time when the "relationship" tends to be raised as a paragon of what is therapeutic, thereby forgetting that pathology is *also* a product of the relationship.
3 *Au fond de l'homme: cela* is the title of the first French edition, which was later reissued under the title *Le livre du ça* ("The Book of the Id") (1963 as part of Gallimard's *Bibliothèque des Idées*, then from 1973 in the *Connaissance de l'Inconscient* ("Knowledge of the Unconscious") collection and finally in the *Tel* collection).
4 I previously used this quote to develop the theme of intentionality, summarized here, in the chapter entitled "Intentionality in Flesh and Blood" in Robine (2004).

Chapter 19

Social Change Begins with Two

"For several weeks", he says, "I've been wondering if I should stop going to therapy, since I feel like I'm not making any progress; I'm going in circles; I'm wasting my time . . ."

"Could you be aware of the way in which you are going about things which keeps you from making progress?"

At the risk of caricaturing and reading into the situation, since I have provided this interaction without any context, let us examine what the psychotherapist might say and what would remain implicit, enfolded in his or her response:

It is clear that if things aren't moving forward, you alone have something to do with it.

It is no less clear that I cannot be to blame and that I put all my skills to work to support your progress,

But I am limited by your resistance to change.

By implicit definition, the resistance is located on the patient's side.

The psychotherapist is an expert in psychic life and, as such, understands aspects of his or her patient's experience to which this patient most likely does not have access.

The psychotherapist therefore has more power and more expertise than the patient,

And is only limited by the limits of the patient's cooperation.

If the patient does not provide access to one or another component of his or her experience, the reason for this should be sought within the patient's resistance and defence mechanisms.

This therapist's concept of human beings includes the idea that we are separate beings, each one responsible for him- or herself. This separation precedes undifferentiation, the integration of experience of what is sometimes called "internal" and "external" . . .

The "Take responsibility for what happens to you" implicit in this therapist's command indicates that this is the individual's responsibility, since the individual precedes the relationship.

The therapist thus adopts an "objectivist" perspective: i.e. that the other is the "object" of the therapist's contributions, skills and expertise.

DOI: 10.4324/9781003515760-23

To understand what a patient says to the psychotherapist, the latter must refer to the way in which the patient considers his or her history – even immediate history. What precedes the patient's statement must be analysed. The aforementioned therapist thus listens to the patient in terms of the self's "personality function" (that is, the therapist listens to the patient say who the patient thinks he or she is), and not in terms of the "id function", which would manifest the "how", perhaps in a stammering, veiled way, a request, a quest, a search for direction for the future, i.e. following the present moment.

We could go on listing a number of other implicit assumptions contained within a simple question from the therapist.

Perls insisted that his patients transform their questions into assertions, since, he maintained, every question contains an implicit assertion. If this working hypothesis is grounded in some truth, it must also be applicable to the therapist. In line with this hypothesis, I myself maintain that every statement made by the psychotherapist – every question addressed to the patient – reveals the map of the therapist's world. It expresses his or her understanding of humans and of the world, of psychopathology and pathogenesis, of change and thus of the way in which he or she intends to inflect the situation.

Questions that may appear quite harmless, such as "What are you feeling?", "When did that start?", "Could this remind you of an episode from your child-hood?", etc. express the psychotherapist's assumptions and prejudices, and thereby reveal his or her perspectives regarding change.

An interview conducted by a psychotherapist involves the simultaneous collection and provision of information. Patients receive this information, even if they are not aware of it. This is why psychotherapists and analysts have long observed that Jungian patients have Jungian dreams, Kleinian patients have Kleinian dreams, etc., and this phenomenon is not limited to dreams, but affects the entire experience.

What then is the information that I wish to transmit to my patients? Do I wish to say, for example, "By revisiting your history, we will find the keys to unlocking change today", "Immediate awareness and the expression of your feelings, emotions and sentiments are crucial to your progress", "You alone are responsible for what you are living", and so on?"

1. Which Reality?

Reality is not a given. Neither is the reality in a therapeutic situation. Reality is constructed. It is a social, relational construction, not the construction of an isolated individual. This difference is substantial, and furthermore it demarcates the dividing line between the constructivist movement and social constructionism, since the latter considers that communication must be understood as a process of constructing social reality, *which is shared among social actors.*

Constructivism, founded by George Kelly in 1955 and largely taken up later by authors such as Maturana and Watzlawick, is an epistemological position that considers that "reality" is fundamentally an "intellectual construct" resulting from scientific preconceptions that one cannot avoid having when one "perceives" and "orders" this famous "real" in order to render it intelligible. The grids of perception and interpretation that a person uses are fundamentally linked to theories, concepts and all the experience that this person has at the moment that he or she questions, investigates or constructs meaning.

Social constructionism, a movement with multiple roots (including constructivism) mainly represented by Gergen and McNamee, extends this constructivist perspective to a certain extent, but at the same time breaks with it by asserting that reality is constructed through relationships, intersubjectivity and dialogue, and not only through the psyche. If we pushed the logic of this epistemology, we could say that there are no "real entities, no facts to know, no systems to understand and no structures or rules to update. There are only speaking, communicating individuals who together build a reality that is born through a process of language" (Vansteenwegen, 1998).

2. Some Consequences for Psychotherapy

Following this logic, each individual's development is either open or closed depending on the terms used in the statements constructed to understand one's experience.

Each sentence that a person pronounces acquires its [provisional] meaning through what follows it – through the "supplementation", to borrow a term from Derrida, provided by the listener in response. The addition made by the psychotherapist only acquires its meaning when the patient supplements the therapist's speech or act by responding, and vice versa. Each interaction is thus both a progressive closure and an opening of potential outcomes.

As psychotherapists, we therefore have an immense responsibility in our choice of words and representations that we use in relation to our patients: in the choice of logic – even implicit – that organizes our thoughts and our response.

Which convictions structure a given therapist? For example, does memory contain traumas or does it invent them? Is a patient the "victim" of his or her trauma or of his or her way of remembering it? Can emotions be "retroflected" and in this way stored? If they are stored, can we do without the fundamental support of the concept of the unconscious? What understanding do I have of temporality? Is the concept of regression relevant to this understanding? Does repetition exist or is it my construction of reality? How can I reconcile a global approach with a theory of polarities? And so on and so forth.

The beliefs conveyed by individuals build their realities, and these realities are maintained through social interaction, which in turn confirms beliefs which are themselves social in their origins. This is true for the average person you pass in the street, for our patients and for ourselves, psychotherapists who maintain our beliefs and our assumptions through our social interactions, our research meetings and our publications.

The words of the patient are assumed to be the reflection of *his* or *her* reality. This argument is rooted in the constructivist school of thought. These words reflect traditions, the cultural community and the system of relations, which is what social constructionism corrects.

These words and representations were certainly constructed through relations, but they *were not* only in the past: they *are* at the moment at which they are pronounced! They are *also* constructed through the speaker's relation to the listener. As a result, gestalt therapy takes one more step thanks to the field perspective: these words *also* refer to the situation here and now, and in this way they bear witness to the specificities of the speaker as well as those of the listener, without being immediately attributable to one or the other on an individual basis.

What could be more quintessential of Gestalt therapy, in short, than this delocalization, this decentring of the individual, this refusal of the primacy of the individual in contacting? My intention here is to extend the entire radicalization initiated by Goodman based on Perls' intuitions.

A few days ago, I noticed a simple, insignificant fact while listening to an interview with a teacher during a radio news broadcast. They were discussing the objectives of the education system and even though the discussion was mostly waffle, the waffle they chose was not entirely innocent. Referring to the national education system, they talked about the plan to train autonomous, responsible individuals. What could be nobler, in short – but in a startling reversal of figure and background, I suddenly realized that I had never heard our educators, teachers and other instructors of young people mention among their objectives the goal of *training individuals capable of creating bonds!* This is not part of the discourse – prefabricated or not – of our era; it is probably not part of the values encouraged by the dominant culture. Individualism is a perverse effect of the development of the individual; I would even go so far as to call it a failure of this perspective since, in my view, autonomy only has meaning within the context of connection.

3.   The Therapeutic Relationship Models Social Change

This social change, which continuously begins with an Other, between two or more, can and should be experimented with during the therapeutic encounter. I would like to mention several supplementary parameters while attempting to define them around three essential characteristics of the self as suggested by Perls and Goodman: spontaneity, the middle voice,[1] and being engaged with the situation.

3.1.   Spontaneity

The psychotherapist's spontaneity – which of course has little to do with reactiveness, impulsiveness or random behaviour elevated to an ethos – is a major component in the make-up of the therapeutic situation. The demand for control has often been imposed on the patient, just as it has been imposed upon all of us at different points in our lives, and has thus contributed to the development of his or her pathology. The encounter of a simple situation, relaxed and yet creative, opens up a space in which one can let go and allows for a certain detachment from the shame of being whomever one is.

This spontaneity is also what brings us closer to the creative powers of a child: curiosity, action, improvisation, play, flexibility, imagination, surprise, risk-taking, encounters with the unknown and the novel, creation, acting, experimentation – important ingredients in the therapeutic relationship according to gestalt therapy.

The self is decentred since, according to Goodman's very terms, it is where the action is. If we felt like playing with the different connotations of the term, I would gladly posit that gestalt therapy is an "eccentric" psychotherapy (as opposed to a "concentric" one, certainly, but also as an incentive to wander around the margins).

3.2. The Middle Voice

In summary, this means being simultaneously active and passive, both sender and receiver in the same communicative act, "both willing and done to", like a child in the situation of a game or an artist in a situation of creation, who have served as a paradigmatic reference in developing our understanding of the self. It is also the principle that is at work in our concept of contact-boundary, as well as in that of creative adjustment since this latter concept implies that in the same operation we are simultaneously transformed by and transforming our environment.

3.3. Engaged with the Situation

There is no self without engagement with a situation, according to the theoretical proposals of our founders. There is much to say about the forms of the therapist's engagement within the therapeutic situation. It seems high time to recognize loud and clear that there is no "neutrality", not even a "benevolent" one, since as soon as two beings are in one another's presence, a process of reciprocal influence is engaged. Of course, influence does not imply that the therapist recommend certain choices to the patient, but it does demand that the processes of introjection be scrutinized and that they perhaps not be as quickly subjected to public scorn, as was the case in certain periods of the history of psychotherapy in general and that of gestalt therapy in particular. Influence does not mean suggestion.

A psychoanalyst, even one of the most orthodox, wields just as much influence as any other psychotherapist, and it would be more than welcome for a number of them to move beyond denial regarding this issue. At the beginning of the legislative debates on the status of psychotherapists, Jacques-Alain Miller insisted to all who would listen that the difference between psychoanalysts and psychotherapists resided in the latter's use of suggestion and placebos. A barefaced denial that suggestion could exist in psychoanalysis! And if by "placebo" we are meant to understand that "it is the relationship that heals, not the substance", then yes! we use a form of placebo, which does not mean "seduction", either!"

4.   A Few Other Aspects of Our Method

In addition to these comments based on the three traditional characteristics of the self, I would like to add a few complementary reflections on certain other aspects of the therapeutic situation and of our concepts that seem important to me for our proposal.

In my view, the caricatured example with which I began this chapter (like other traditional techniques of a certain type of gestalt therapy, such as the reappropriation of projections or the dialogue with an empty chair) often falls under what I would call a "premature individuation" based on a "premature responsibility".

If we adopt a field perspective and accept the hypothesis of "contact as the first experience", with which our founding text opens, this means that we have to set off again, methodologically speaking, from an initial undifferentiated situation – the famous "creative undifferentiation" that Perls borrowed from Friedlander, which characterizes the field as a whole. The idea that the feeling or experience of the moment is immediately attributed to the person who expresses it falls under a theoretical prejudice to which gestalt therapy opposes another theoretical prejudice: it is the product of the situation – and therefore a co-production – that involves undertaking individuation based on a progressive, provisional differentiation, by distancing the intervention of the self's personality function as much as possible (which is to say, in more definite terms, relatively little!). Indeed, the self's personality function is quick to draw on prior representations of "the person I know I am", which by the way is more "the person I know I was", and to look for a confirmation of these representations in the present moment. This confirmation can only close off any possible opening to what is new, and thereby allows nothing on the scale of a change rooted in recognizing the experience lived here and now. As a result, this premature individuation is no longer a process of individuation but rather a fixation with this illusion that we call "individual".[2]

What I am living here and now is the product of our encounter, of the situation, and as such, says as much about me as it does about you. Of course it is also the product of my personal history, or more precisely of my current representation of my history, but this is so rich and complex that all sorts of experience make it up, including the most contradictory.

It is the present moment, the resonance between the form[3] of the present moment and certain components of my own history, which will awaken these elements and mobilize them in the form of memories or learned processes. If I claim sole responsibility for what I am living, I deny both you and your impact on the situation and on my experience. The self does not precede contact. It creates contact and is created in contact, in the middle voice. Lévinas clearly established the difference between "being responsible" and "taking responsibility", and I invite us all to return to this distinction in order to nuance this issue. Each of us is totally responsible for the other but, in spite of this, we do not always have to "take responsibility for" the other. Of course, the potential contribution of Lévinas' work to the theory and practice of psychotherapy would deserve more ample development.

Another example: a certain type of manipulation that we – often wrongly – call *awareness*, since it is the immediate, implicit awareness of the field. It is forms of work on awareness, the psychotherapist's questions or comments that willingly plunge the patient into shame. The invitation to be aware of a certain posture, gesture or process leads many patients to associating this with an experience of reproach: "I shouldn't . . . I should be aware (i.e. more controlled), I'm not the person I should be, etc." A number of patients have opened my eyes to this issue.

The problem of shame constitutes an exceptional occasion to work within a field perspective. Shame is indeed an experience that fundamentally isolates us, traps us in a mouse hole, tries to remove us from the other's view; it is experienced as something arising from within oneself. However, shame does not exist without an Other – the shamer – who generates this experience or re-opens the wound. The appearance of shame in the therapeutic situation is therefore a chance to refocus what is abusively or prematurely experienced as personal, intimate or intrapsychic at the interactional level. Moreover, the therapist must be in touch with his or her own modalities of defence or release from shame. As a result, to return once again to the interaction that I mentioned at the beginning, it is clear that the patient who tells me that he isn't making progress thereby stimulates my own shame, even if I remain unaware of it. It is no less clear that I may use "any means possible" to avoid feeling shame about my inadequacies or incompetence, and that my "favourite" means of defending myself consists in willingly ridding myself of this problem by plunging the other into shame, thereby creating the illusion of my superiority and expertise.

Instead of doing this, if I understand and recognize my defence system, and dare to open up when it activates during my contact with this patient, the shared creation of which links us together, this seems to me to denote another understanding of the world, of the encounter and of the human relationship. It denotes another vision of society, founded on connection, mutual influence, interdependence and solidarity, joint construction.

5.   Conclusion

If I believe that only contact and encounter can be constitutive and transformative, and that a subject only exists in and through contact, encounter and dialogue, an initial task is required of me, as a psychotherapist, and inevitably leads me to apply this understanding of humanity to myself: what I have enjoyed telling myself about identity for more than sixty years is fundamentally a representation of contacts, situations and encounters *and* of the way in which this experience has been metabolized within me, knowing that this integration of experience is itself a pursuit of contact, not a solipsistic experience. What we call "self" – which, as Perls reminds us on a number of occasions, is a function that belongs as much to the organism as to the environment and thus cannot be assimilated into "me" – this self, therefore, is what organizes these experiences. As a result, "I" am only a co-organizer of experience, whichever experience may be involved.

I believe that a successful psychotherapy is a process in which clients change their assumptions, change the conversational modes in which they are involved, change their narrative . . . in short, change paradigms. This transformation takes place on the occasion of a psychotherapist who can offer conditions for making this possible, since he or she has been able to undergo this transformation and him- or herself, and thus to be present in encounters.

Context: This essay, and the following chapter, deal timidly with the social dimension of gestalt therapy. I've always kept my distance from conferences and assertions about the impact of our approach on society, which seem to me to be overly pretentious, but I sincerely believe that the methods of contact that are implemented, unfolded and explored in the course of our sessions can have a repercussion on the ways in which each person encounters his or her everyday life, in the hope that a certain transduction will take place. This text is a slightly revised version of lectures given to the Société Française de Gestalt, at the 2005 Kiev Gestalt Therapy Congress and various other places.

Notes

1 Perls and Goodman use the expression "middle mode", which is a mistake since Greek grammar uses the term "middle voice" to designate this grammatical category.
2 This aspect is developed in further detail in my study entitled "Intentionality in Flesh and Blood", to which I refer the interested reader (see Robine, 2011b)
3 See in particular the concept of "morphic resonance" in the work of Sheldrake (1985).

Chapter 20

Some Social Implications of Gestalt Therapy

What I want to sketch, introduce and especially to discuss is not as much about the various commitments that one or another person may make in society or the social functions that we may exercise through our roles as about all the social consequences linked to the *form* of therapy that we propose. I would thus like to expand upon a topic that I already began to discuss under the title "Social change begins with two".[1]

I consider that the succession of contacts established between the therapist and his or her client, and their organization into a relationship, regardless of the approach used, contributes to modelling social relations and anchoring clients within the social fabric. American pragmatism effectively demonstrated that the means define and colour the ends, so the results obtained will be modelled upon the methods employed. I hypothesize that a therapeutic experience lived through gestalt therapy will not have the same effects as a therapeutic experience lived with a Lacanian psychoanalysis, a Jungian psychoanalysis or a bioenergetic analysis. I am also aware that within a single approach, we may observe major variations linked to the therapist's person, system of values, concept of human beings and own personal history.

I would therefore like to limit my remarks to what seems implicitly or explicitly linked to theory and method, and to draw upon the ancient wisdom of the Stoics, especially Epictetus,[2] who urged us to know how to distinguish "what depends on us from what does not depend on us".

Let us take this a bit further. The title – and the content – of a book by James Hillman, a well-known Jungian psychoanalyst, struck me when it came out in 1992: "We've had a hundred years of psychotherapy, and the world's getting worse."[3] It would seem that gestalt therapy is not the only one to have a limited impact! The title of this book could even imply that psychotherapy has had a negative impact, if we wanted to establish a cause-and-effect relationship! I don't know whether the world is getting worse as a result of psychotherapy, but I believe that psychotherapy may contribute to this problem by introducing several perverse effects, particularly egotism, disengagement and disempowerment.

DOI: 10.4324/9781003515760-24

Egotism

Egotism is defined rather paradoxically in gestalt therapy, since it refers to an excessive reference to oneself, excessive functioning in ego mode, which results in a slowdown of interaction at the boundary, excessive control, insufficient spontaneity, letting go to the point of cutting contact. This definition is paradoxical because our authors present this excessive functioning in ego mode in the chapter that they devote to "Losses of ego-function". This implies that this excessive control of contact through the ego-function is not the result of a choice one has made . . .

Through his teaching, Isadore From brought to light how psychotherapy – and Gestalt therapy in particular – created a sort of artificial neurosis by focusing on questioning and the development of the ego-function: "What do *you* want? What do *you* feel? What are *you* aware of? What do *you* choose?" These repeated questions of course centre the patient on him- or herself. According to From, this egotist neurosis is the gestalt twin of transference neurosis, which is created by the analytical situation as a tool to elucidate infantile neurosis. The dissolution of the egotist neurosis, like the dissolution of the transference neurosis, are meant to signal the end of the treatment. From willingly admitted that he saw a limit to these two approaches, which were not always able to bring the process to a close – in other words, to dissolve the tools that they had created to be able to operate.

It seems undeniable that gestalt therapy does not have a monopoly on the egotizing effect of therapy. A number of authors have highlighted the culture of individualism and the culture of narcissism that have developed quite substantially over the past few decades. As an example, here are several lines from Christopher Lasch's famous study, "The culture of narcissism":[4]

The principal allies [of the psychological man of the twentieth century], in his struggle for a sense of personal equilibrium, are not priests, proponents of autonomy, or captains of industry like the self-made men of an earlier era, but therapists.

(p. 23)

A little later, he continues:

Therapy has established itself as a successor to rugged individualism and religion, not that the "triumph of therapy" has become a new religion in itself. In fact, therapy represents an anti-religion, not because it concerns itself with rational explanations and scientific techniques of healing, as its practitioners would have us believe, but because modern society "has no future," and therefore pays no attention to anything not immediately relevant to its needs.

(p. 17)

And again:

Even when therapists talk about the need for "love" and "meaning" or "purpose", they define these concepts only in terms of meeting the patient's emotional needs. It scarcely occurs to them [. . .] to encourage the client to subordinate his needs and interests to those of someone, or something, outside of his own dear self. "Love" as self-sacrifice or humility, and "meaning" or "purpose" as submission to a higher loyalty, these are the sublimations which the therapeutic sensibility experiences as intolerable oppression, as an offense against common sense, and as a threat to the individual's health and well-being. To free mankind from such primitive notions as love and duty is the mission of post-Freudian therapies, particularly of their popularizers and disciples, for whom mental health means the removal of inhibitions and the immediate gratification of impulses.

(p. 48)

Humanism, which certain gestalt practitioners claim to adhere to, is one of the last avatars of individualism. Many have reproached Perls for his "gestalt prayer", often considered an egotist manifesto: "You are you, and I am I. I am not in this world to live up to your expectations, and you are not in this world to live up to mine. If by chance we find each other, it's beautiful. If not, it can't be helped." Today it may indeed be ironically interpreted as an invitation to indulge in sense-less egotism, if we consider it within our contemporary social and cultural context. However, as certain authors effectively demonstrated: "Within the context in which Perls formulated his 'prayer' (1960s America), where people were no longer able to separate themselves from attachments that weren't working, these assertions took on a curative value."[5] In our contemporary society, where each of us is invited to follow our own path, to take care of ourselves "because we're worth it", these values and methods are firmly entrenched and extensively exploited by the mer-chants of personal development.

Far be it from me to deny the importance of individuation, differentiation, and therefore even a necessary, desirable egotism. Every human being has to build up knowledge that is balanced between his or her need for identity differentiation and his or her need for connection. The pathologies of narcissistic experience are one of the forms of failure to construct a dialectic between these two opposing neces-sities: they result from favouring the identity aspect to the detriment of belonging.

Disengagement and Disempowerment

With all due respect to Christopher Lasch, we need to understand what is happen-ing to us; nothing is more nerve-racking than remaining without meaning – it is even the very definition of terror – and nothing is more reassuring than having a response. The causalist response is the most accessible and offers cheap reassur-ance. Through their method, the different therapies incite us to look for the causes in our personal history, in childhood sexuality, in genograms and cross-generational transmissions, in family secrets, in interactional structures, in the language that structures our exchanges, in genes and biological heredity, in personal or social traumas, etc. The phenomenological psychiatrist Arthur Tatossian[6] linked autonomy and its opposite, heteronomy:

> Every therapy [. . .] presupposes the heteronomous conditioning of the experience or behavior that it targets, and it matters little whether this heteronomy is exerted by some imbalance in neuronal synapses, by a particular organization of the unconscious or even by some misfortune of Dasein.

The relation that we establish with what we set forth as causes is a heteronomous relation, as if the causes were foreign to experience and systematically portrayed as "mitigating circumstances".

It is doubtless in response to this excessive disempowerment generated by the psychoanalyzing approach being rendered more and more commonplace, and a poorly assimilated psychoanalysis that led Perls (with his trademark artificiality) to insist on responsibility: "Take responsibility for what you feel; take responsibility for your emotion; be aware that you are the one who has created this dream, this situation, this conflict, this symptom, etc."

While working on the concept of "situation", I came across the work of a Spanish philosopher from the first half of the 20th century, José Ortega y Gasset. One of his phrases – "I am me and my circumstance"[7] – held my attention insofar as it integrated the issue of the situation and circumstances within the contours of identity. During an intervention in Spain, I was able to ask colleagues about this philosopher that I hadn't known existed before then, and about this phrase of his. I learned that it had since then been decontextualized and absorbed into everyday language, a bit like Sartre's famous "Hell is other people".[8] For example, when an employee was late to work because of traffic jams and met with criticism, he could easily use the excuse: "I am me and my circumstance." We are clearly quite far from the philosophy developed by Ortega y Gasset!

In our team of Gestalt trainers, we very quickly sensed and then observed several potential negative effects when we began to radicalize the reference to field perspective in training gestalt therapists. If it is offered as an alternative to the intrapsychic reference, it may cause personal empowerment to fade into the background behind the situation or context, according to the modalities evoked regarding Ortega y Gasset.

However, in work that falls within a field epistemology, we know that everything that is present has an impact on contact, including various elements that are not always taken into account. The therapist's explicit recognition of his or her conscious portion of influence, defences, potential projections, countertransference and investments or counterinvestments introduces a dynamic of responsibility linked to the situation, from instant to instant.

The Reduction of the Social to the Psychological

The popularization of psychoanalyzing discourse has sometimes contributed to reducing social issues to psychological ones: class struggles or the demands of trade unions are chalked up to unresolved problems with authority or with the father figure, the complexity of superimposed links within small communities (such as our own) is theorized in terms of incest, violence in rough neighbourhoods is ascribed to a superego deficit or the integration of the law, war is viewed in terms of projective identification and political engagement as a need for reparation, etc. I consider this reduction of the social to the psychological to be a sign of arrogance, as if we were sure to hold the keys to understanding the world.

In his day, Max Pagès invented the concept of "stump theories" (*théories moignon*) to refer – within a discipline – to the presence of simplified representations of neighbouring disciplines that are "incorporated into the dominant theoretical system and necessary for it to function".[9] This way of working characterizes the systems of thought that aim to dominate the intellectual landscape, and psychoanalysis is not alone in employing it. It represents a discipline's need to picture neighbouring disciplines, since it is impossible to build a psychology or a metapsychology, for example, without at least a representation of the social on the one hand and the biological on the other. In our own discipline, we have thus witnessed the appearance of a "neurogestalt", just as we saw a "systemic gestalt" or an organizational gestalt bloom around Cleveland and among this centre's followers. Recognizing the importance of neighbouring approaches seems absolutely essential to me, but other modes of recognition may exist beyond total or partial engulfment. It should, however, be noted that retreating within one's discipline is just as sterile and sectarian: the discipline will quickly take on an almost religious way of functioning, or even a fundamentalist, religious communitarian approach.

The link between the instinctive and the sociopolitical has always been difficult to theorize. In other words, how can we resolve the dilemma between the individual's spontaneity and the social structuring described by Freud in *Civilization and its Discontents*?[10]

To develop his personal response to the questions of human malaise, Freud attributed the incompatibility between individual needs and social obligations to this "discontent with civilization", and stated that the only solution was for the individual to functionally adapt his or her needs to social requirements. Introjection thus became the dominant mode by which social rules were interiorized in order to make them become "superego".

But this did not stop Freud from writing, in a letter to his friend Pfister:[11]

Thus discretion is incompatible with a satisfactory description of an analysis; to provide the latter one would have to be unscrupulous, give away, betray, behave like an artist who buys paints with his wife's house-keeping money or uses the furniture as firewood to warm the studio for his model. Without a trace of that kind of unscrupulousness the job cannot be done.

Is there a disconnect between his public position and his private choices, or is this a paradox, or even an oxymoron?

We are familiar with Perls' first response: he offers his concept of the aggressiveness of deconstruction as necessary for survival and for physical and existential growth.

The second part of his response: by positing that organism and environment are inseparable, every situation becomes a function of this contextualized relation, and no longer an alternative.

Third response: It is precisely at this border that creative adjustment may take place, as an alternative to the dilemma set up by Freud in terms of having to choose between either repression/inhibition OR sublimation.

What is the creative adjustment offered by gestalt therapy?

Perls and Goodman agreed with the criticism levelled at psychoanalysis in their time, accusing it of adapting itself too much to society. They did not deny the necessity of the adaptation by which the individual is transformed to meet social requirements, but they added creation as an inseparable element: adaptation that creates (and is not only creative), that transforms the environment in a single act, in the middle voice.

What Depends on Us

In my view, the exceptional strength of gestalt therapy – at least when it is practiced within a reference to the field paradigm – resides in its ability to apply three combined modes of action, three areas of work with our patients.

Identity Construction

The first area of work involves identity construction and individuation. Gestalt therapy is of course not the only psychotherapy to have an impact on the deconstruction and reconstruction of identity. Nonetheless, its reference to the unity of experience, its use of work by immediate awareness, its tools that allow it to link the personality function to lived experience in the here and now, making room for the id of the situation, etc. all lend a particular force to our method.

The attention paid to moments of presence opens the door to what is "really" lived, beyond representations, fixations, ideals and other introjects.

Access to the World Lived by an Other

As a result of his or her particular mode of involving – or unveiling – the self, the gestalt therapist is in a modality of appearing in the eyes of his or her client that leads the client to establish the gestalt therapist as an Other and thereby to think about otherness. Closing oneself off through egotism or remaining indifferent to the experience of the Other, both of which are so characteristic of our contemporary society, are also confronted. Contacting and being contacted are occasions for measuring the impact on an Other and the Other's impact on ourselves which, beyond reflexivity, contributes to the construction of identity and progressively constitutes the other as an Other – in other words, this allows us to learn *idem* from *ipse*, sameness from differentiation, and the radical alterity of the Other.

Intersubjective Relationship, Connection, Belonging . . .

The very awareness of the Other's existence through contact work allows the intersubjective distance to be reconstructed. The field perspective in which the gestalt therapist's ethics and epistemology are rooted opens the way for the process of relational ebb and flow – the movements that enable the shift from undifferentiated to differentiated and vice versa. It is also what is sometimes called the "fusion/separation" dialectic, along with its procession of consequences such as dependence/autonomy, influence and manipulation. The experience of phenomena inherent to the therapeutic relationship – not reduced to mere transferential phenomena – make up a testing ground for the connection and belonging that are so lacking in our societal context.

As I see it, gestalt therapy's social plan takes shape through these three working directions and requires investment from all three, which cannot be dissociated from one another. It is clear that, according to the phases of therapy and the process that is unique to each therapeutic dyad, one or another of these modes will be put into practice and temporarily favoured. However, the specific character of the gestalt approach requires these three ingredients to be integrated, without claiming that the therapeutic action is limited to these directions. Choosing these focal areas is itself a societal and a political choice.

An Essential Social Act: Recognition

For several generations, a great number of psychotherapists and psychoanalysts, with Winnicott at the forefront, have stressed the importance of the demand for recognition that is at the heart of the therapeutic demand. The suffering, symptoms and psychopathological modes of existence would gain from being more often considered in light of this issue and not only in terms of the vagaries of the libido or of defences against anxiety. Axel Honneth,[12] a German philosopher who succeeded Jürgen Habermas in the wake of Hegel, demonstrated how social evolution is constructed through a series of real or symbolic struggles in which the individual does not aim so much to remove or reduce his or her adversary as to be recognized by him or her as an individual. He thus revisited the mechanisms of personality formation as they were illustrated by G.H. Mead, a stalwart of American pragmatism, and Donald W. Winnicott, a psychoanalyst, to offer his sociohistorical and psychosocial analysis. The frameworks that he proposes strike me as being more than relevant to consider within the psychotherapeutic context. The bond of recognition is built through love, law and solidarity. Self-confidence is built through the recognition obtained by love. Self-respect is built through the recognition based on law: legal recognition. Self-esteem is built through the recognition provided by social solidarity.

Honneth takes up the question that Winnicott grappled with his entire life: "Through what interactive process do a mother and her child manage to separate themselves from this state of undifferentiated unity, in order to learn to accept themselves and love themselves as independent persons?"[13] This recognition refers to

the double process by which one simultaneously liberates and links the other person emotionally. [. . .] [It is not a consideration] of the other on a cognitive level but rather in the sense that one shows affection for the other and thereby accept his or her autonomy.[14]

It is thus through the love of the Other that one builds self-confidence.

At first glance, what Honneth calls "legal" recognition appears to concern the psychotherapist only marginally. However, the author follows in G.H. Mead's footsteps "to consider that the social recognition of legal rights has its corollary in the development of one's capacity to depend on oneself as a morally responsible person",[15] and it is through this recognition that this person may acquire the capacity to understand his or her acts as a manifestation of his or her own autonomy, respected by all. Legal recognition also means the right to exist.

Lastly, self-esteem is built through solidarity. "The extent to which I actively ensure that the other's specific qualities, insofar as they are not my own, manage to develop determines whether our common goals will be achieved."[16] The community of values and of shared ethics is at the forefront. Its absence generates shame, humiliation and wounds.

These three forms of recognition are at work in the therapeutic relationship. Deficits in one or another of these forms of recognition constitute disturbances that lead certain people to come knocking at the doors of our offices. We know that these intersubjective conditions make up the conditions necessary for individual self-realization, and the philosophy of contemporary gestalt therapy, like its methodology, has evolved in parallel with the social and psychological developments of the contemporary world.

Gestalt therapy has no roots: it has a rhizome, which is a sort of subterranean arborescence that does not order influences into a hierarchy but rather opens the way to complexity. It is neither psychoanalytical nor phenomenological nor Reichian, nor is it a branch of pragmatism or gestalt psychology; it is not even a harmonious combination of all these seeds: it is dialectic, pulled between all these forces, since the original gestalt therapy explicitly claimed to be biopsychosocial. Even if our practice essentially develops in the two-person colloquium held between a gestalt therapist and his or her client, gestalt therapy's political, social and psychosocial plan may be incarnated at every minute of work which is held together by contact.

Just as in gestalt therapy, dependency is just as important as autonomy; so-called infantile spontaneity is just as important as deliberate character; conflict and aggressiveness are just as important as love and tenderness; pre-genital sexuality is just as important as genital sexuality; the false dichotomy between the individual and society does not hold up. Of course, the complexity of the therapeutic situation leads us to choose certain working methods while social intervention professionals will choose others, but our entire philosophy, our ethics and our methodology implore us to aim for contact between humans and the world, in order for the support, belonging and solidarity that directed the establishment of the therapeutic relationship to be extended into everyday life. But let's not be too optimistic . . .

Context: A small step further in developing some of the themes addressed in the previous chapter. Much remains to be done . . . This text was used as the basis for numerous lectures in conferences held in Eastern Europe in 2010 and 2011.

Notes

1 J.-M. Robine (2005), "Le changement social commence à deux", *Gestalt Journal*, no. 29, December.
2 Epictetus (1964), *Entretiens*, in *Les Stoiciens*, La Pléiade, pp. 808 ff.
3 J. Hillman and M. Ventura (1992), *We've Had a Hundred Years of Psychotherapy, and the World's Getting Worse*, Harper San Francisco, translated into French in 1998 with the title *Malgré un siècle de psychothérapie, le monde va de plus en plus mal*, Ulmus Company, London
4 C. Lasch (1979) *La culture du narcissisme*, Paris, Champs-Flammarion, 2006.
5 Salonia G. (2010), "Changements sociaux et malaises psychiques", in G. Francesetti (ed.), *Attaques de panique et postmodernité*, Bordeaux, L'exprimerie, 2010, p. 52. See also S.F. Crocker (1983), "Truth and Foolishness in the 'Gestalt Prayer'", *The Gestalt Journal*, vol. VI, no. 1, Spring; French translation "Vérités et sottises à propos de la prière gestaltiste", Mini-bibliothèque de GT No. 112, IFGT 2010.
6 *Pratique psychiatrique et phénoménologie* (abridged, provisional version), typescript for a seminar of the Bordeaux psychiatric phenomenology research group. Undated (1970s), unpublished.
7 This turn of phrase was selected by the *British Gestalt Journal* as the title of an interview that they published in their journal. Interview translated and published as Chapter 7 of J.-M. Robine (2004), *On the Occasion of an Other*, Bordeaux, l'exprimerie.
8 Sartre, during an interview in 1964, wrote: "'Hell is other people' has always been misunderstood. People thought I was saying that our relationships with others were always poisoned, that relationships were always hell. Actually, I meant something completely different. I wanted to say that if relationships with other people were twisted and vicious, the other couldn't be anything but hell. Why? Because deep down the others are what is most important in ourselves, for our own awareness of ourselves. When we think about ourselves, when we try to understand ourselves, deep down we use knowledge of ourselves that others already have; we judge ourselves using the means that the others have – that they have given us – to judge us and ourselves. Whatever I may say

about myself, the other's judgment always enters into it. Whatever I may feel about myself, the other's judgment enters into it. This means that if my relationships are bad, I make myself completely dependent on the other, so I am indeed in hell. And there are a number of people in the world who are in hell because they are too dependent on the judgment of others. But that does not in any way claim that one cannot have other relationships with others; it only points out how singularly important the others are to each of us."

9 M. Pagès (1990), *L'analyse dialectique: propositions*. Conférence introductive au Colloque de Spetzès. Document interne du Laboratoire de Changement Social, Université Paris VII.

10 *Le malaise dans la culture*, 1929, *Œuvres complètes,* tome XVIII, Paris, PUF 1994.

11 Freud, letter to Oskar Pfister, cited in P. Rieff, *The triumph of the therapeutic: uses of truth after Freud*, Chatto & Windus, London, 1966, p. 107

12 A. Honneth (1992) *La lutte pour la reconnaissance*, French translation Paris, Ed. du Cerf, 2000.

13 A. Honneth (1992) *La lutte pour la reconnaissance*, French translation Paris, Ed. du Cerf, 2000, p. 121.

14 A. Honneth (1992) *La lutte pour la reconnaissance*, French translation Paris, Ed. du Cerf, 2000, pp. 131–132.

15 A. Honneth (1992) *La lutte pour la reconnaissance*, French translation Paris, Ed. du Cerf, 2000, p. 144.

16 A. Honneth (1992) *La lutte pour la reconnaissance*, French translation Paris, Ed. du Cerf, 2000, p. 157.

Chapter 21

What I Believe . . .
and What I Believe I Believe

Introduction

I've often developed the idea of decentralization or relocation to clarify the epistemological rupture introduced by Perls and Goodman in their theory of the self. I originally borrowed it from a 1968 interview Paul Goodman had with a student named Glassheim who was preparing his PhD thesis. This idea seems to cover many characteristics of gestalt therapy's approach:

> *Paul Goodman*: [. . .] There is no soul . . .
>   *Eliot Glassheim*: A decentralized soul?
>   *Paul Goodman*: . . . the soul is wherever the action is, that's where the soul is, where the action is.
>   *Burton Weiss*: That's a nice way of saying it, decentralized soul.
>   *Paul Goodman*: Yeah, the functional soul. We have that as a doctrine in Gestalt therapy – what do we call it, the principle of dominance or something or other. That is, in any situation there gets to be a natural hierarchy of functioning, relevant to the situation. It is dominant. [. . .] Nothing else in the behavior will make sense, if you leave that out, because that is the dominant factor. This is Kantian, too, by the way! His Synthetic Unity of Apperception.
> (Glassheim, 1973, p. 207)

1. Decentralizing

The self is not something located deep within the human being; there is no true self or false self as Winnicott and other psychoanalysts theorized; the self is action; the self is contact with the world. I am the action I take; I am what I express; I am how I act; I am the contacts I establish. What we call the self's personality function is the system of representations that I construct over time through my actions, my contacts and my experience of the world. This personality function is therefore made up of beliefs forged over time; it structures the rhetoric of *what I believe*. What I believe is a construction, although it is certainly based on experience, but it's also a fiction: a representation that suits me and contributes to the image I have

DOI: 10.4324/9781003515760-25

of myself, sometimes idealizing it and sometimes devaluing it. That's why – and in this respect it is faithful to Goodman's conviction that the soul (or self) is where the action is – there may be a difference between "what I believe I believe", through my system of representations and verbalization, and "what I believe", which also reveals itself through action, in the unformulated or the implicit, immersed in situations, and which may reveal major differences.

This gap – which I recognize in myself and I notice in each of us, and which I refer to here as the difference between "what I believe" and "what I believe I believe" – is important to become aware of. The consistency that we all try to construct between the different levels of our experience involves continually narrowing this gap. It is also one our supervisors' responsibilities to remind us of this distance, from their outsider perspective, and help us bring it into the realm of awareness.

2. Situating

About ten years ago, I suggested to the gestalt community that we build on the concept of "situation". This concept seemed to provide a major insight into the field stance, which is so difficult to grasp when you don't want to convert the field into a tangible, objectifiable thing. Understanding that we simultaneously create and are created by situations opens up the possibility of thinking outside an individualistic, isolationist logic to focus on another kind of presence. I am created by the situation of my presence to the other, and at the same time I am the creator of this situation.

Some of my friends and colleagues who are gestalt therapy theorists built on this concept. This was the case of Dan Bloom (2013), for example, who discussed the notion of "situated ethics". For us, situated ethics is an ethic of gestalt psychotherapy. "It is pointless, therefore, to attempt to deal with any psychological behavior out of its sociocultural, biological, and physical context", wrote Perls, Hefferline and Goodman (I, 6). But a few lines later they add:

The fact that the gestalt has specific observable psychological properties is of capital importance in psychotherapy, for it gives an autonomous criterion of the depth and reality of the experience. It is not necessary to have theories of "normal behavior" or "adjustment to reality" except in order to explore.

We are therefore confronted with two dimensions of ethics: an extrinsic ethic and an intrinsic ethic. Extrinsic ethics refers to the shared morality that defines good and evil, and right and wrong. It is an ethic of content. Intrinsic ethics is the behaviour that connects one person to another and even structures how we are with one another. It is an ethic of the contact boundary of *this* therapist and *that* client, which exposes *that* suffering he is experiencing. It is therefore an ethic of the process: of the construction of the gestalt in the situation.

When socio-political, economic, cultural, racial, moral or religious considerations act as references in the situation, extrinsic ethics take precedence over intrinsic ethics and situated ethics, and the process of gestalt therapy can be jammed up by it.

Of course, it is not always easy for the gestalt therapist to make this distinction and set aside his or her preconceptions, values and beliefs, as required by the phenomenological approach. There is a tension towards this *epoché* that can be expected of each of us.

This difference between the two ethical references clarifies issues when, for example, a transgression committed by a psychotherapist towards one of his patients must be investigated, such as in the case of sexual abuse. If we refer to extrinsic ethics, which in some countries is known as a professional code of ethics, the transgression will be discussed in terms of misconduct and breach of professional rules. If we refer to intrinsic ethics – situated ethics – we will frame it in terms of a serious lack of awareness on the therapist's part, a lack of awareness of the issues and barriers to the therapeutic process that he has thereby generated, a disturbance of the personality function that points to a confusion between functions and contexts, a disturbance in the definition of the relationship and of what may emerge in contact-boundary, and so on.

3.   Thinking

Thinking is an act and, like any other act – even a spontaneous one – it contains an element of deliberate choice.

As strange as it may seem, it took me a number of years to become fully aware that my thoughts were not something that *came to me* or fell into me as might any object in my environment. Everyday language induces this implicit representation: "I just got an idea", as if I were just the custodian: the person who receives the idea. I could also say I tried to "drive this idea from my mind"! I "thought" . . . or at least I could say so, although it would have been more accurate to say that "I was thought by my thoughts", using the passive form of conjugation. And thoughts "that came to me", related to my culture, my knowledge, my values, my introjections and whatnot, could impose themselves on me like obvious truths.

This went on until one day I realized that certain concepts, which I had been using to think, had a sort of relative relevance: they could be useful to me in some contexts but prove toxic in others. I was thus confronted with the opportunity to *choose* how to think, to choose what to think, and to choose what type of knowledge was relevant to my experience. Of course, I don't always *feel* like the manufacturer of my thoughts, and sometimes I still experience my thoughts *as if they came to me*. But I can choose my words, I can choose my concepts, and I can distance myself from (gestalt therapy would say "alienate") those who alter my ability to contribute my services to the development and creative adjustment of the people I support.

For a clinician and to explain (and I mean *explain,* not *understand*) a patient's behaviour, concepts such as "polarity", "regression", "repetition" and many others might very well be relevant. For me, as a gestalt therapist, these concepts can also be toxic and pollute my contact with the other.

I'll take the example of "repetition". Diagnosing repetitive behaviour means focusing on what doesn't appear new to me and separating it from the overall experience; this means ignoring the novelty of the situation and everything that might be different in what the other is letting me see. It means forgetting the insistence of this *petition,* which is renewed and which neither I nor others have probably wanted to hear until now. What, then, is this insistence on the contact boundary? What is this closure on my part towards perceiving it?

Are my modes of thinking oriented towards development, change and openness to the thrust of the id function of the self and the implementation of the creative adjustment that would result from it? Or are they oriented towards tracking down fixations, revealing deficits and looking for a primary causality, which is certainly reassuring but oh-so-illusory?

What I believe is expressed through my language. My language structures my dichotomies, including what Perls and Goodman call "false dichotomies" such as "mind/body", "self/outside world", "childish/mature", "biological/cultural", "conscious/unconscious", "spontaneous/deliberate", "love/aggression", etc. Language is also what structures my implicit and explicit representations, my fantasies and my ideals, my values and my ethics, and my beliefs.

4.   Constant Indissociation and Differentiation

My language, my questions and my affirmations do not come from me and me alone. They are the product of the contact that develops with the other: they are a co-construction. As proof of this, all you need to do is try telling a story (or describing the plot of a film or novel, or a chapter of your personal history) to several different people, and measure the differences between successive retellings. These differences reflect the contact boundary: what is woven between the other and myself in the present moment. This is another way of thinking about the foundational character of the field.

There are many different ways of contemplating the concept of field. They all have their merits, and they all have roots in various physical, psychosocial, biological, philosophical and other conceptions of the field. Among the various options, I choose the one I believe is most relevant in the context of my practice of gestalt therapy. For me, the field is not a "thing": a physical or objectifiable entity. It is not the "context", either, especially since it often only involves the environment – "my" or our environment, not the indissociable organism/environment field, as Perls and Goodman define it. Objectifying expressions such as, "There's this or that in the field" or "It's in the field" don't make sense to me. "The" field does not exist: all that exists is the field of a given being and of what makes up its experienced environment.

The field I refer to is a field *of experience*. It consists of everything that is relevant to a subject at a given moment. Of course, I know there may be elements or factors in my living space which I am not aware of but which may nevertheless contribute to my experience of the moment. I would say they are not part of my field of consciousness, but they can be part of my field of experience. Certain aspects of my experience being experienced can be brought to my consciousness through certain modalities, and psychotherapy is one of them.

What makes up the field for me at a given moment is structured by the situation, at the same time as I contribute to structuring the situation. In the situation of psychotherapy, I co-structure the situation together with the other, and it is sometimes difficult to predetermine what will belong to him, what will belong to me and what will belong to both of us. That's why I think it's important to agree on starting with a hypothesis of non-differentiation and uncertainty. This methodology opens up to the experience of the present moment and thereby helps us set aside prior representations of identity, prior knowledge of what I call "myself", and preconceptions. New knowledge of self, new contours and new insights may emerge from the work that develops from this undifferentiated field, and they in turn will have to be deconstructed by the next contact, and so on. This leads me to consider that what we call "identity" is a fiction, like a story that I like to believe in: a "what I believe I believe" that I most definitely need to ensure my historical continuity but which hinders my openness to the novelty offered by each now.

5.   Apparatus

However, the therapeutic situation does not arise randomly from a purely "spontaneous" encounter between beings who co-create the event. Psychoanalysis has imposed the concepts of "framework" or "setting" and "rules", which have connotations I find hardly suitable. Others rely on the concept of technique, which I accept if it refers to *techne* in its original meaning referenced by Heidegger: "the bringing-forth of the true into the beautiful" (Vaysse, in Zarader, 2002). I prefer to think in terms of an "apparatus" – which to my mind implies and contains these concepts – to refer to one of the structural elements of the situation. Michel Foucault (1977) provided what is probably the most precise definition of this concept:

> What I'm trying to pick out with this term is [. . .] a thoroughly heterogeneous ensemble consisting of discourses, institutions, architectural forms, regulatory decisions, laws, administrative measures, scientific statements, philosophical, moral and philanthropic propositions – in short, the said as much as the unsaid. [. . .] The apparatus itself is the system of relations that can be established between these elements.

Later he says:

> I said that the apparatus is essentially of a strategic nature, which means assuming that it is a matter of a certain manipulation of relations of forces, either

developing them in a particular direction, blocking them, stabilizing them, utilizing them, etc. The apparatus is thus always inscribed in a play of power, but it is always linked to certain coordinates of knowledge which issue from it but, to an equal degree, condition it. This is what the apparatus consists in: strategies of relations of forces supporting, and supported by, types of knowledge.

This detour via the concept of apparatus – in addition to being of interest in discussing what others prefer to call a framework, rules or setting – also allows me to express my conviction that psychotherapy is not and cannot not be a truly dual and dialogical I–Thou relationship. In my view, a true dialogue implies parity and mutuality. Unlike many relationships of everyday life, the contact here is structured by an apparatus that has a function as a third. The apparatus is a third pole of the relationship which structures, orders, limits, contains and organizes choices. This apparatus is not a co-creation, although certain forms through which it manifests itself are produced by the protagonists and the situation they develop together. This apparatus is selected and implemented by the therapist, and it serves to inflect the situation and place data into the process. When a true I–Thou relationship is created – a relationship as described by dialogical philosophy – it may be considered an indication of a change as the end of the therapy draws near.

6.   Experiencing

For a long time, I believed and taught that the essence of psychotherapy laid in the construction of meaning, and that for many of us, the therapist's task was to guide his client through restructuring the meaning of what he had experienced or was currently experiencing. Today I have a different vision, which is both broader and narrower. Today I consider the concept of experience – experience lived in the current situation – to be crucial. I do not believe in the therapeutic power of a single meaning. I think that, in essence, experiencing in a contact situation is what can open up an integrated assimilation, new representations, new adjustments and new meanings. After all, every experience contains many ingredients other than meaning; experience is a kind of reservoir for unformulated elements that take on various forms and meanings depending on the circumstances, situations and people involved. Of course the absence of meaning can cause anxiety or even terror; meaning soothes anxiety, sometimes cheaply, and I accept this necessity, but it seems important not to set a fixed meaning – it should be accepted as transient. Gadamer emphasized the inexhaustible nature of the experience that constitutes meaning: "It's never finished" (Gadamer, 1960, p. 84). Setting and resetting the experience into motion allows new meanings to be created. I like to quote the philosopher Alain who wrote, "Ideas, even true ones, become false as soon as one is satisfied with them" (1968).

Experiencing in the current situation implies being open to the present moment and to encountering its novelty. Many currents within psychotherapy and psychoanalysis like to reference the Socratic method (also known as maieutics). As much as the teachings of Socrates transmitted by Plato may have greatly contributed to my intellectual training, I now believe that the Socratic approach is diametrically opposed to the approach of gestalt therapy. The term "maieutics" is derived from the Greek word for "midwifery": the science of delivery. This technique involves thoroughly questioning the other person in order to make him deliver his knowledge, which he holds hidden away within himself.

This is the same type of logic employed by Freud who, to explain the work of the analyst, used the metaphor of an archaeologist who uncovers and reveals buried remains (Freud, 1905a). However, shortly before his death, in his work entitled *Constructions in Analysis* (Freud, 1937), he opened up the perspective of construction, or more precisely that of reconstruction based on these remains.

Perls and Goodman frequently mention the "discovering-and-inventing" pairing (e.g. Perls, Hefferline and Goodman, 1951, X, 6). *Dis-covering* means revealing what was buried, implying that the material was already there, present and accessible to those who knew how to look for it. This is similar to maieutics, since nothing can be delivered unless the person already has a baby inside her. This approach mainly focuses on what is already there, revealing the past and what has been repressed; it is an approach that delves into the archives of the person; its conduct is structured by looking into a rear-view mirror. *Inventing* involves a creative process: it is the act of conceiving something new. This approach is therefore consistent with the creative adjustment that gestalt therapy provides as an objective and a means of therapy. It means driving while looking forward, ahead of oneself ("standing ahead of oneself" is the translation of the term "presence"), facing the next.

7.   Several Elements of the Position I Believe In

7.1.   Openness

By this I mean openness to the other's experience, openness to the unknown, openness to difference and openness to contact.

It includes the openness to do what is necessary to free oneself of what could be: what it would have been better to do. It involves considering that the patient or client, in the circumstances and situations that he has experienced, did the best he could to survive and adjust with the resources of his field.

7.2.   Non-Judgement

Non-judgement avoids placing the client in a situation of shame. Shaming, humiliating, and expressing contempt, anger and other similar affects are attitudes that can reveal my frustrations, my own unfinished situations, and my need for additional therapy and supervision.

7.3.   Engagement, Involvement and Disclosure

One of the characteristics of the self, when activated, is being engaged in the situation: engaged in the co-construction of the current figure. The therapist's presence cannot be considered neutral, even if he is invited to set aside his own systems of values and references. His involvement can go as far as a measured level of self-disclosure.

Unfortunately, I have often found that, for a number of gestalt therapists, exercising with reference to field perspective means talking about oneself in resonance with what one's client has experienced, without overly questioning oneself on the merits and limitations of this exposure. In a field perspective, since the therapist is part of the client's current environment, it is certainly interesting when the therapist can evoke how he is affected by the presence or processes implemented by the client (Robine, 2004, 2007). The difficulty lies in assessing the relevance of this disclosure and ensuring that it is applied to serve the figure that the client is constructing (and not any narcissistic or seductive aims on the part of the therapist), within the limits of the contours of his experience in the here and now of the situation. I have only rarely perceived situations in which there is a real interest in narrating one's own personal experience and history. Self-disclosure by the therapist is a material that should be used to approach the targets and the emerging intentionality of the client in the situation.

7.4. Tenderness

I do not like the term compassion, which is often used to refer to the feelings we have when confronted with the suffering of others. Despite its use by certain Eastern philosophies, for me it retains a connotation of condescension, commiseration and pity that I do not like. I am also quite ambivalent towards the concept of empathy, which involves some form of identification with the other and leads to "objectified self-enjoyment", as shown by a masterful study that was one of the first to approach this concept (Worringer, 1911). Instead, I prefer tenderness. It is an affective involvement that engages my sensitivity, my fragility and my emotional understanding. It's what enables alliance and of course what unfolds within the relational system defined by the therapist, establishing and safeguarding the rules that govern how our profession functions (Delourme, 1997). Involvement and distance must be able to go hand in hand. Tenderness provides a pre-reflective background for the connection with the other. It represents an emotional home base for the expression of affects, including aggression and hatred, which may need to explore and express themselves in both transference and the current relationship.

7.5. Asceticism of the Now

The here and now has long been one of our favourite slogans, to the point where we willingly introject it into our clients. It is certain that the now is all that exists, and that this now contains memories and expectations. These days, it seems to me that the now is much more a sort of asceticism for gestalt therapists: a focus that allows them to keep their attention on the process, contact and its variations, the experience being constructed at the boundary, and the situation. It is the awareness that *this* client is talking to *me*, and that while he is telling me about his past experience, he is simultaneously describing his immediate experience, with each one illuminating the other.

7.6.   Faith

At the heart of my position, there is faith. My conception of faith, as Goodman describes it throughout the pages of *Gestalt Therapy* (Perls, Hefferline and Goodman, 1951) and his other writings, revives its original meaning, before the various religions took it by force. "Faith is knowing, beyond awareness, that if one takes a step there will be a ground underfoot." Or: "Absorbed in the actual activity, he does not protect the background but draws energy from it, he has faith that it will prove adequate." And: "This feeling of being ready for anything is perhaps what theologians call faith."

7.7.   Desire or Eros?

Lynne Jacobs (2010) brought an interesting article by the philosopher John Riker (2009) to the gestalt community's attention, entitled "The Life of the Soul: An Essay in Ecological Thinking". In this text, in which the author prefers to discuss the soul but also makes room for the self, in his Kohut-esque conception, he posits the alternative between Desire and Eros.

> The soul properly engaged with its essential life is not the Desiring Soul but the Erotic Soul. Desire seeks to consume the world, to transform what is other into what is mine. Eros loves the world and reverences its beauty. It wants to merge or join with the beauty of its objects, not consume them.

Faced with a conception of gestalt therapy that has all too often focused on need and desire, in this sense a worthy successor of psychoanalytic thought which gives pride of place to lack and castration, it opens a path which, instead of narrowing experience down to the satisfaction of needs, opens experience and complicates it. It's about going beyond the stage of the desiring soul to achieve an ethic of Eros: being human and learning to be with the beauty of what *is*, not what might be or what could have been. Psychotherapy can legitimize its roots in an aesthetic position.

7.8.   Ethics

An ethic based on the concept of need and desire undoubtedly relies on neuroscience to better explain (here it's about explaining, not understanding) the individual's psychic functioning. Psychotherapy thus takes a scientific orientation in which an expert bases his position on knowledge about the other, and works using reproducible techniques. Even if such a form of medicalized psychotherapy may prove undeniably useful in treating mental illness, we are still quite far from a phenomenological stance which urges us to set aside constituted knowledge and the culture of uncertainty (Staemmler, 2003a, 2006b), or the choice of "no longer knowing" (Blaize, 2001). I believe in gestalt therapy as applied philosophy (Miller, 2004) and even as an aesthetic, since we work towards the formation of forms and creative adjustment (Robine, 2006b).

In *Agamemnon*, the Greek tragedian Aeschylus introduced the expression *pathei mathos*, which is often translated as "learning through suffering" and which I would translate as "what is learned through what is felt". This formulation gave rise to the concept of "pathic", which was extensively developed by phenomenologist clinicians such as Von Weizsäcker, Straus or Maldiney (1991). Maldiney in particular pointed out that "it is through the pathic that the being knows himself: not in an objective, thematized way, but through what affects him". Feeling and experiencing are the source of the openness of self and the contact with the world that structure forms of presence – the psychotherapist's and the client's alike.

Context: *Although this text was written a few years before "On the Good Use of Incoherence", it is the expression make of similar concerns: how to make what we do correspond to what we say we do, and how to what we say we do correspond to what we do. My experience of supervision, both as supervisor and supervisee, reveals gaps, gulfs that are sometimes impressive ravines . . . so exciting to discover. Closing lecture at the Ukrainian National Congress of Gestalt Therapy, 2011.*

Chapter 22

Intimacy, Encounter, Tenderness . . .

Since the origin of the human being, at least since we have written traces of their thoughts and feelings, and whatever the forms of evolution of the human condition, the theme of love and all its variants occupies a privileged place. After "The Song of Songs" of the Bible, the poems of ancient Egypt, the tales of *One Thousand and One Nights*, Plato's "The Banquet", and the poetry of the troubadours or the romantics, I will not assume that our contemporary contributions will finally put an end to our reflections, our doubts, our comments on this theme.

Wittgenstein (1921) included *love* in his list of "false words" (*ein falsches Wort*), that is, those which, when they are used, one does not know what they are talking about. Would that not be the case with many words, if not with all? I know of many words that we use in our microcosm without really making sure that we are talking about the same thing, for example *contact, field, self, aesthetics* . . ., and this is even the case with concepts of more restricted scope such as *introjection, contact-boundary*, etc.

When I was a young gestalt therapist, one of my first patients, after two or three years of weekly sessions, arrives one day for our meeting with a defeated look on her face, obviously in a state of anxiety close to panic. The only thing she can say to me is: "I NEED to know if you love me." Struck and unbalanced by the unexpectedness and urgency I perceive in her request, rightly or wrongly I decide to answer, "Yes, I love you . . ." and after the time of a short breath, I add: "I love you . . . not like a father, not like a lover or a friend, not like a brother!" Was I wrong, was I right to address such a direct response? Was I wrong or right to add those precisions that were able to define my feeling only by what it was not?

In the 1970s and 1980s, the European beginning of the therapies that were then called "new therapies", the rebellion was led by the psychoanalytical orthodoxy. One of the favourite arguments of its ayatollahs: Gloria's filmed session with Carl Rogers during which, to this patient who told him, "Gee, I'd like you for my father!" he dared to answer, "You look to me like a pretty nice daughter" (Shostrom, 1965). This polemic had impregnated me and was undoubtedly part of my background when I responded to this young woman. It is difficult to imagine today the scandal created by such an answer, which manifested, according to this rear guard, a total absence of consciousness, neutrality and mastery of counter-transference (*sic*).

DOI: 10.4324/9781003515760-26

This, at the time, was considered grounds for excommunication, or its oft-heard civil equivalent, "If this is so, we have nothing to talk about to each other" (*sic*).

I liked how the confusion between levels of experience had been exposed by Virginia Satir, the famous humanistic family therapist, in a workshop I attended. She liked to make physical contact with the patients she was working with: a hand on their shoulder, a support on their back and other supportive gestures. To a psychoanalytic psychiatrist who criticized her for eroticizing or even sexualizing the relationship in this way, she asked wryly, "Sir, do you know the difference between a hand and a penis?"

At a time when psychotherapy – and gestalt therapy – claims to add the precision of "relational" to its name, I feel the need to consider some of the ingredients of what constitutes the in-between of what happens when two human beings come into the presence of each other. Referring to love, as it happens regularly, does not suit me. Neither the psychoanalytical reduction of the relationship to a displacement called transference, nor the new-age idealization proposed by pop-psychology or the hard-discount mysticism on sale in the news stands or workshops, help me to name or explain the variety of phenomena that emerge from this "face to face".[1] Thus, I would like to evoke some reflections about certain concepts which, of course, refer to specific experiences that can be undergone in the therapeutic relationship: intimacy, tenderness, encounter.

Intimacy

Intimacy is what is contained in the depths of the being. The suffix *-imus* (*intimus*) added to *in* or *intus* (inside) indicates in Latin that it is a superlative: that which is *most* interior, or *very* interior. When we speak of intimate thoughts, intimate notebooks, "intimate parts" (so-called calls in my language – French – and in the English language "private parts"), we are speaking of what is completely private and generally hidden from others or, in any case, will be offered to the sight only of a few.

But "intimate" is also a modality of *being-with* since we also speak about intimate relations. Would it be paradoxical to use the same word to designate an experience that is essentially interior, solitary, and an experience of contact and great proximity?

In the first meaning of the "most interior", however, the other is already very present in spite of his/her absence, since one tries to hide one's thoughts, one's notebooks, one's sexual organs, from the other! Could one suppose that what is "most interior" gives rise to the necessity of a sharing, to the need to abolish the dichotomy inside/outside, even if only episodically? Would the intimacy with the other give a reason of being to the innermost, and for the innermost would it make exist the need to be fertilized? To be intimate with another means that I have opened to him/her the access to what I consider as my "innermost". Intimacy thus refers to a state of feeling *and* to an interpersonal event; it refers to private *and* public, hidden *and* revealed, and intrapsychic *and* relational issues.

Can "Intimate" Qualify the Therapeutic Relationship?

It is undeniable, from now on, that there is a closeness, an intensity in what is called the therapeutic "relationship". In everyday life, intimacy is a relationship of reciprocity, of openness to the other and of mutuality in accessing the "innermost" of each other, but is this the case in this very specific situation in which the functions are specifically defined.

Magda Denes, one of the first gestalt therapists, and at the same time an existential psychoanalyst, has created a little parable that highlights the attributions of each:

> One evening, a pig and a hen are shipwrecked. They find themselves alone on a desert island; wet, hungry and miserable. They spend the night in hopeless vigil while a cold wind blows. As the sun rises the hen shakes herself and says, "Look, we might as well make the best of it. The least we can do is have breakfast. Let's have ham and eggs." The pig looks at her, thinks for a while, arches an eyebrow and replies: "But Madam, from you that is a contribution, from me it is a commitment."
>
> (Denes, 1982)

This emphasis on the specific attitudes of both protagonists is sometimes denied by some contemporary writers who insist on reciprocity, mutual transformation, idealizing Buber's I–Thou as the gold standard. They may forget that Buber himself, in his famous dialogue with Carl Rogers in Ann Arbor, Michigan, in 1957, had already warned against this oversimplification in the course of their dialogue.

> A man is coming to you for help. The essential difference between your role in his situation and his is obvious. He comes for help to you. You don't come for help to him. And not only this, but you are *able,* more or less, to help him. He can do different things to you, but not help you. And not this alone. You *see* him, *really* [. . .] as he *is.* He cannot, by far, cannot *see you.* [. . .] You are of course a very important person for him. But not a person whom he wants to see and to know and is able to. [. . .] He is not interested in you as you. It cannot be. You are interested, you say so and you are right, in him as a person. This kind of detached presence he cannot have and give.
>
> (Buber, in Kirschenbaum, p. 49)

And Buber insists:

> [. . .] You have necessarily another attitude to the situation than he has. You are able to do something that he is not able. You are not equal and cannot be. [. . .] I see you *mean* being on the same plane, but you cannot. [. . .] I am not speaking now about your feeling but about a real situation.
>
> (Buber, in Kirschenbaum, p. 49)

Their dialogue was about how psychotherapy, and thus in particular the existential-humanistic psychotherapy represented by Carl Rogers, could build on the famous I–Thou model introduced by Buber. Rogers declared himself to be a strong believer in this word-principle and, paradoxically, it was Buber who moderated his ardour. Later, the dialogic gestalt therapy movement, particularly promoted by Gary Yontef, Richard Hycner and Lynne Jacobs, insisted on the need to differentiate the "I–Thou attitude", the "I–Thou moment", the "I–Thou relationship" (Yontef, 1993, 2021; Hycner, 1991, 1995). But I am still reluctant to include the concept of "relation" as it stands in our theoretical apparatus and to organize a theorization based on it. If, indeed, it is possible to accept that "the relationship" can have therapeutic virtues, it is impossible for me to hide the fact that the relationship is also the foundation of all forms of psychopathologies. By limiting themselves to the slogan, would it be a way, for its supporters, to avoid clearly identifying what, of the relationship, can be a resource for development and what, by its toxicity, can be at the origin of various psychopathologies? Hence, my incessant quest for a more precise understanding of what, in a relationship, could have a therapeutic impact!

In order to try to understand if this can help us to shed light on the outstanding question, to evaluate the relevance of qualifying as intimate what happens in this in-between, as unbalanced as the therapeutic situation, let us explore a little more this idea of "relationship".

The Encounter

When the encounter begins to settle, it becomes a relationship. When the encounter settles into a relationship, otherness is lost. This shocking proposition of the French philosopher François Jullien is at the heart of his latest writings (Jullien, 2013, 2016, 2019). The other is no longer other since she has allowed herself to be assimilated by me. "The encounter has buried itself fled – beneath the relationship", he writes (2019).[2] To encounter, indeed, requires a gap and it is this gap that allows the other to emerge as other and to contact. Empathy – or inclusion – if they can be considered as modalities of understanding the other, could not thus, in my eyes, be considered as modalities of *contact* since they abolish, of course temporarily, the difference and the gap.

It is through the encounter that I can discover the other. In the encounter, I experience the unexpected, I can be astonished. I can even be surprised by the other, even unbalanced, bewildered. Distraught? Does this mean that I do not feel "taken over" by the other? Could this be where the contrast between the relationship and the encounter lies, because in the relationship something of me is assimilated by the other and something of the other is assimilated in me? But it is through surprise and astonishment that I can evolve. In our relationships, do we succeed in introducing renewed encounters, surprise and astonishment, gaps and imbalances? Intimacy is the fruit of the meeting, of the encounter, and the "relationship" is often a way to avoid intimacy. To have accumulated a "knowledge about" the other is not to be intimate; to have such an "experience of the other" that there are no more surprises is not to be intimate because there is no more gap, perhaps even no more true *presence to*; there is only mastery, assimilation, undifferentiation, when inclusion becomes chronic in low-grade intensity.

The encounter is shock, clash, it is violence, even if it is soft and tender. Precisely because it maintains the gap. Because none of partners is master of the encounter. And the intimacy that it creates is not an intimacy of knowledge; it can be intense, implicit and ephemeral. Sometimes, at the end of a session, I feel tears in my eyes. It is not what the patient has told me that upsets me, it is not his or her story, his or her theme, his or her suffering, but the way something has opened up in him/her, and the way something has opened up in me, which gives both of us the impression that we have reached the most essential, most of the time unnameable, *intimus*, the most interior, as the etymology recalls. I probably would not have said anything about myself in this meeting but I also feel joined at the "most interior". And my "most within" can only exist because it has opened itself to your "most within". This intimacy is of course ephemeral, metastable and that is what makes it transformative. The chronic, the habitual hardly contains any seeds of evolution.

This experience of intimacy as a moment lived together in the situation could perhaps correspond to what some gestalt therapists call – wrongly, in my opinion – "full contact". The original theory spoke of *final contact*, and *final* was to be understood not as the *end* of the sequence but as the *finality*, that is, that moment when what had emerged during the fore-contact in terms of direction of meaning can find its realization, its concretization in the situation. This moment when, sometimes, therapist and patient fall into each other's arms is often called "full contact" whereas it is only very rarely a "final contact" since it was probably not the gestalt that had emerged and that had gradually been elaborated in the sequence. *Moment of intimacy* thus seems a more appropriate denomination, especially as it would avoid the impression that a final contact had just been experienced.

The original theory of gestalt therapy does not often make use of the concept of relationship nor define it. The whole theory is based on the concept of *contact*, which cannot be superimposed on or substituted for that of relationship; it is joined by that of situation, which offers a context in which contact can unfold and thus positions psychotherapy. However, contemporary trends use and abuse "the relationship", without defining the contours of this concept. Contact and encounter are certainly not synonymous, since contact designates any operation that articulates a subject and its environment, whether human or not. And the meeting is a form of contact even more restricted, since it implies the interhuman face to face, the presence and the mutual opening.

Tenderness

To speak now of *tenderness* could probably belong to another writing. However, it seemed necessary to me, after having briefly introduced the theme of love before evoking that of intimacy and encounter, to return to the affective experience at the heart of any link, whatever it may be. To speak of love or friendship to name what develops in the therapeutic relationship seems to me to be abusive because "love" does not only designate a certain type of feeling, for example affection, but also a certain type of mutual bond. Thus, I would not call love the feeling that someone can have for someone else without there being reciprocity. This is why I think *tenderness* is one of the feelings that a therapist can experience towards his/her patient, that I feel towards my patients, my supervisees or students, and I do not need this feeling to be reciprocal.

This feeling is not a posture, but a progressive construction that can become a chosen attitude,[3] a slow opening linked to the increasingly fine perception that I can have of all that this patient has been able to elaborate in order to adjust to the people who constituted his environment and created with him the circumstances of his existence. The theory of gestalt therapy invites us to look at the implementation of any symptom, of any psychopathology, as a creative adaptation, as the most relevant construction that the person has been able to elaborate with his environment at this particular moment of the situations that were repeated with insistence.

Unlike some therapists who have addressed the question of tenderness in the therapeutic relationship, I do not expect reciprocity of this feeling here and I do not consider it legitimate to consider or expect tenderness as reciprocal: it seems to me essential that my welcome can be felt as an opening to all forms of experience, emotional experiences and modalities of their expression on the part of my patient. It is essential that anger or rage, affection or admiration, envy or jealousy, hatred or resentment, disgust or eroticized seduction, boredom or attraction can manifest themselves just as freely, whether these affects, moreover, turn out to be embedded in a transference dynamic or seem to be inscribed in the reality of the encounter and of its evolution. Tenderness does not seek to encompass the other, nor to be encompassed by him/her, nor to possess him/her.

Freud (1905b) considered tenderness as an eroticism which would have been diverted from its sexual finality. He suggested that the normal character of the sexual life associates tenderness and sensuality in its tension towards the object. Thus, for him, the entanglement of tenderness and sensuality is the guarantee of the good functioning of sexuality.

"Unfolding" Tenderness

And if tenderness, separated from libidinal impulses and sensuality, does not seek the satisfaction of the sexual goal that characterizes them, should we then consider that the tenderness of the therapist towards his patient would be an effect of the sublimation of his sexual impulses? Why not? This would be an opportunity to make room for sublimation again, a modality of loss of the ego-function outlined in the founding text (PHG, 1951) but mostly forgotten by later theorists.[4] Let us recall that for Freud (1905b), sublimation allows the satisfaction of needs and desires following usual social standards which established what could be appreciated or not. PHG (1951) correct this proposal by considering that sublimation is a direct but imperfect satisfaction of the same need (450). The interpretations that PHG propose, completely inscribed in a post-Freudian conception of sexuality, do not convince me very much especially since by insisting on the "imperfect" character of the satisfaction of the need, they model implicitly what could be the "perfect satisfaction".

But since I mentioned sublimation here, one of the somewhat forgotten inflexions of contact, the question of tenderness could also incite us to look at the other modality of regulation of repression evoked in the same Chapter 14 of PHG: the *reaction-formation*. It too is often forgotten or neglected by today's clinicians, perhaps because we would only see this concept in terms of its intrapsychic appearance, but yet it seems to be very much a constituent of what is known as a person's "character" and thus clearly a field effect. In the reaction-formation, the security offered by the repression of unacceptable impulses – unacceptable by the subject or by his environment – does not seem sufficient. To the uncertain repression will be added, in order to reinforce it, an additional covering operated by a reversal into its opposite. Tenderness could then turn out to be the reaction-formation of rejection, indifference, malice, antipathy, aggressiveness, cruelty, even sadism. Of great importance is the therapist's personal therapeutic journey, during which his/her motivations for this professional choice are usually explored in depth. Experienced clinicians have often found that repressed impulses, when covered by a reaction-formation, can ooze out without the holder's awareness and thus prove harmful to the patient.

Tenderness could also be one of the forms of expression of *pity*, or of its more socially valued form, *compassion*. I admit that I have for a long time been critical of pity, attributing to it a foundation sometimes in a form of exaggerated sentimentality, sometimes a defensive conversion against rejection or disgust, and no doubt many other "good" reasons for dismissing it from my benchmarks for understanding. Until one day, while reading, I came across the following analysis in a novel by Stefan Zweig (1939):

There are two kinds of pity. One, the weak and sentimental kind, which is really no more than the heart's impatience to be rid as quickly as possible of the painful emotion aroused by the sight of another's unhappiness; that pity which is not compassion, but only an instinctive desire to fortify one's own soul against the suffering of another. The only one that counts, the unsentimental but creative kind, which knows what it is about and is determined to hold out, in patience and forbearance, to the very limit of its strength and even beyond.

(p. 176)

In this second form of pity described by Zweig, I can find not only a root to the tenderness I can feel in the face to face with my patients, but also a strength to hold on, to stand firm (to contain, to support, to hold back, to maintain, to hold on . . .) which constitutes in my eyes one of the characteristics of the therapeutic attitude

I have had the opportunity to consider as essential (Robine, 2004, pp. 240–241). It is curious to note that historians of the French language trace the etymology of *tendresse* to the family of Latin verbs *tenere* (to hold) and *tendere* (to tend) (see Rey, 1992, p. 2099).

The *Most-Inside* Shared by Tenderness

Tenderness is therefore a non-passionate form of affection, among other reasons probably because it excludes any form of possession and does not expect any reciprocity from the other, nor does it demand anything in return. Some would willingly modify my formulation to say that it is a non-passionate form of *love* but, as I mentioned above, I prefer to reserve love to designate the fruit of a long-term work between two beings, in the same way that it is necessary to differentiate between *to love* and *to fall in love*. It is also undoubtedly what had led Françoise Dolto to propose the term of *aimance* (Dolto, 1981, p. 333).

What Sylvie Consoli, a dermatologist and psychoanalyst, says about tenderness ("to be tender") will not surprise the gestalt therapist who, since gestalt therapy has existed, has never ceased, in various forms, to push clinicians to abandon the pseudo-neutrality or the distant coldness that has been a dogma for decades:

> I attach great importance to the capacity of a psychoanalyst to let himself be touched by a patient, not only in the usual sense of this term ("to be touched"), but also in that of letting himself be tenderized by the other. That is, to deform, to change. As if any change of the patient [. . .] would pass through the capacity of the analyst himself to change with his patient and to keep the imprint of this change throughout his life as an analyst and even throughout his life in general . . .
> (Consoli, 2003, p. 19, my translation)

It is noteworthy that Consoli uses the French word *s'attendrir*, which means to feel tenderness and to show one's tenderness, while all French–English dictionaries propose only "to be touched" as a translation for this French word.

Can we dare to be tender? Dare to encounter the other, dare to abolish momentarily the border between inside and outside? Dare to respect not in reference to any code of morality but as recognition of the validity of her experience, of his difference, of her creation. When the contact with the other is not based on lack – and therefore on need or desire – and when it does not seek to possess, to fill, at the risk of brutality and abuse to obtain satisfaction, a possibility is opened so that it is the encounter in itself that is the finality.

Opening a space for the expression of tenderness in the therapeutic relationship is at the same time opening a space for pleasure, and even shared pleasure. The awareness that is created in the cognitive domain alone is not embodied and is likely to be ephemeral. After more than half a century of a distanced and cerebral conception of the therapeutic situation, the affect, which is the basis of any encounter, the sensation and the sensitive (*aesthesis*), the corporeality of the lived experience are creating a more and more affirmed place:

> Contrary to what the Freudian technique prescribes, the pleasure that the therapist experiences in his exchanges with the participants is necessary for change. It is not harmful, nor is it a suspicious element that must be measured out, accepted with reluctance and a guilty conscience. It is the motor of change.
>
> (Pagès, 1977, p. 36, my translation)

Psychotherapy is above all a situation, a work situation, certainly, but also an encounter situation since it is the contact and its analysis which are at the heart of the face to face meeting. Most of the contemporary psychotherapies want to be, under various forms, relational. The study of intimacy, which has opened us up to one of its components, tenderness, can lead us to take a different look at the divide that separates the proponents of an intrapsychic, or even individualistic, paradigm from the supporters of a more relational perspective such as that offered by the field theory. Indeed, we have seen that "intimate" designates what is "most inside" but also what can link two beings and we have seen that "at the most inside of oneself (*intimus*), it is the Other who discovers himself there" (Jullien, 2016, n.p.). To be intimate with an Other means that I have opened him to my "innermost". This intimacy does not reduce the gap since for there to be an encounter, there must be a gap. As for there to be contact. It is necessary that the other is always for me a strangeness. Thus, the concept of intimacy could be a concept of reconciliation between the two paradigms by putting in evidence that one cannot exist without the other. Of course, the intimacy evoked in the context of the therapeutic situation is an intimacy of the encounter and not of the relationship.

A few words from Nietzsche will be my provisional conclusion:

> We always end up being rewarded for our good will, our patience, our fairness, *our tenderness towards the stranger*, due to the fact that the stranger gradually reveals itself and comes to offer itself to us as a new and unspeakable beauty: this is its gratitude for our hospitality.
>
> (1882, § 334, italics mine)

Context: *I don't like using the concept of "relationship": too wide, too vague. Of course I know that a relationship can be healing; however, I also know that every psychopathology has been created by relationships. So, step by step, I try to explore some components of the therapeutic "relationship" which could narrow our focus and contribute to unfold and understand what happens in this specific face to face. Originally a lecture at the New York Institute for Gestalt Therapy, it became this article, which was published in French in* Cahiers de Gestalt-thérapie, *no. 46, 2022, and in English in* Gestalt Review, *vol. 27 no. 2, 2023.*

Notes

1 I deliberately write "face to face" here without the hyphens, thus following the choice of Kurt Martin, a commentator on Levinas who, after reminding us that hyphens have the function of uniting or even confusing terms that face each other, insists that they must, according to Levinas's wish, be absolutely distinguished (Martin, 2016, pp. 422–423).

2 All citations from French authors not officially translated into English are mine.

3 In social psychology, Rosenberg (1960) highlighted the three essential components to define an *attitude*: an affective component, a cognitive component and a conative component (behavioural intentions).

4 I can assume, however, that the Polsters' (1973) introduction of their concept of "deflection" is a behavioural avatar of sublimation. They describe it as "a maneuver for turning aside from direct contact with another person. It's a way of taking the heat off the actual contact" (89).

References

Agamben, G. (2006), *Qu'est qu'un dispositif?* Trans. from Italian. Rivages-poche, Payot, Paris, 2007

Alain (1930), *Propos I*, 12 July, Bibliothèque de la Pléiade, NRF, 1956

Alvim Bothelo, M. (2004), *Experiência estética e Corporeidade: fragmentos de um diálogo entre Gestalt-terapia, Arte e Fenomenologia*, Brasilia (Thèse de doctorat, Université de Brasilia)

Aristotle (1922), *On Generation and Corruption*, English trans. Oxford (Book 1, ch. 6, §3) (*Traité de la production et de la destruction des choses*, Librairie Philosophique de Ladrange, Paris, 1866 (Livre 1, ch. 6, §4))

Bachelard, G. (1923), *Préface* à Martin Buber, *Je et Tu*, Aubier, Paris, 1969

Bailly, A. (1894), *Dictionnaire Grec-Français*, Hachette-Paris, 16th edition, 1950

Bakhtin, M. (Voloshinov V.N.) (1929), *Le Marxisme et la philosophie du langage*, French translation, Minuit, Paris, 1977

Balint, M. (1959), *Les voies de la régression*, Payot, Paris, 1972

Baranger, M. and Baranger, W. (1961), La situation analytique comme champ dynamique, French trans. in *Revue Française de Psychanalyse*, vol. XLIX, Nov.–Dec. 1985

Barwise, J. (1989), *The Situation in Logic*, CSLI Publications, Stanford, CA

Barwise, J. and Perry, J. (1999), *Situations and Attitudes*, CSLI Publications, Cambridge

Bergson, H. (1934), *La pensée et le mouvant*, 22nd edition, PUF, Paris

Bernard, M. (1976), *L'expressivité du corps*, J.P. Delarge, Paris

Binswanger, L (1930), *Le rêve et l'existence,* French trans. Desclée de Brouwer, Paris, 195

Binswanger, L. (1947–55), *Introduction à l'analyse existentielle*, French trans. Ed. de Minuit, Paris, 1971

Binswanger, L. (1947–57), *Discours, parcours et Freud*, French trans. Gallimard, Paris, 1970

Blaize, J. (2001), *Ne plus savoir – Phénoménologie et éthique de la psychothérapie,* L'exprimerie, Bordeaux

Blaize, J. (2005), Les "co" de la coconstruction, *Cahiers de Gestalt-thérapie*, no.18, L'exprimerie, Bordeaux

Bloom, D.J. (2003), "Tiger! Tiger! Burning Bright": Aesthetic Values as Clinical Values in Gestalt Therapy. In M. Spagnuolo-Lobb and L. Amendt (eds) *Creative License: The Art of Gestalt Therapy*, Springer, New York, pp. 63–77

Bloom, D.J. (2005), A Centennial Celebration of Laura Perls: the Aesthetic of Commitment, *British Gestalt Journal*, vol. 14, no. 2

Bloom, D. (2013), A Piece of a Continent: The Situated Ethics of Gestalt Therapy. In G. Francesetti, M. Gecele and J. Roubal (eds), *Gestalt Therapy in Clinical Practice – From Psychopathology to the Aesthetics of Contact.* Franco-Angeli, Milan (French trans. *Psychopathologie en Gestalt-thérapie*, L'exprimerie, Bordeaux, pp. 131–145)

Bourriaud, N. (1993), Le paradigme esthétique. Revue *Chimères*, no. 21, winter

Bourriaud, N. (2001), *Esthétique relationnelle*, Les Presses du Réel

Braque, G. (1948), *Cahier (1917–1955)*, Maeght, Paris, 1994

Brentano, F. (1874), *Psychologie du point de vue empirique*, Aubier, Paris, 1944

Brentano, F. (1914), *On What Is Continuous in Philosophical Investigations of Space, Time and the Continuum*, Croom Helm, London, 1988.

Broustra, J. (1996), *L'expression, psychothérapie et création*, ESF, Paris

Broustra, J. (2000), *Abécédaire de l'expression*, Erès, Ramonville St Agne

Brusset, B. (1988), *Psychanalyse du lien – La relation d'objet*, Le centurion, Paris

Buber, M. (1923), *Je et Tu*, Aubier, Paris, 1969

Buci-Glucksmann, C. (2003), *Esthétique de l'éphémère*, Galilée, Paris, 2003

Castel, R. (1973), *Le psychanalysme – L'ordre psychanalytique et le pouvoir*, MasperO, Paris (republished by Champs-Flammarion 10/18)

Chazal, G. (1997), *Formes, figures, réalité*, Champ Vallon, Seyssel

Clément, C. (1990), *La syncope, Philosophie du ravissement*, Grasset, Paris

Colli, G. (1982), *Philosophie du contact, Cahiers posthumes II*, Trans. from Italian by P. Farazzi, Editions de l'éclat, 2000

Collins, R. (2004), *Interaction Ritual Chains*, Princeton University Press, Princeton

Consoli S. (2003), *La tendresse*, Odile Jacob, Paris

Crocker, S.F. (1983), Truth and Foolishness in the "Gestalt Prayer", *The Gestalt Journal*, vol. VI, no. 1, spring (French trans. *Vérités et sottises à propos de la prière gestaltiste* Mini-bibliothèque de GT no. 112, IFGT, 2010)

Delcò, A. (2005), *Merleau-Ponty et l'expérience de la création – Du paradigme au schème*. Philosophie d'aujourd'hui, PUF, Paris

Deleuze, G., (1968a), *Différence et répétition*, PUF, Paris,

Deleuze G. (1968b), *Spinoza et le problème de l'expression*, Minuit, Paris

Deleuze, G., (1969a), *Logique du sens*, Les éditions de Minuit, Paris

Deleuze, G. (1969b), M. Tournier et le monde sans autrui. Appendix to *Logique du sens*, Minuit, Paris

Deleuze, G. and Parnet, C. (1977), *Dialogues*, Champs-Essais Flammarion, Paris, 1996

Delisle, G. (1998), *La relation d'objet en gestalt-thérapie*, Les éditions du Reflet, Montréal

Delourme, A. (1997), *La distance intime – Tendresse et relation d'aide*, Desclée de Brouwer, Paris

Denes, M. (1982), Existential Approaches to Intimacy. In M. Fisher and G. Stricker (eds) *Intimacy*, Plenum Press, New York, pp. 141–158

Dewey, J. (1933), *Art as Experience*, Capricorn Books, New York, 1993

Dewey, J. (1938), *Logique, la théorie de l'enquête*, PUF, Paris, 1993

Dolto, F. (1981), Aimance et amour. In *Au jeu du désir*, Le seuil, Paris

Dossmann, P. (2000), Le complexe de Cyrano – Un séminaire sur la honte avec Jean-Marie Robine. In Clinique de la honte, *Cahiers de Gestalt-thérapie*, no. 7

Dubet, F. (1994), *Sociologie de l'expérience*, Coll. La couleur des idées, Seuil, Paris

Dufrenne, M. (1953), *Phénoménologie de l'expérience esthétique*, 2 vols, PUF, Paris, 1992

English, H.B. and English, A.C. (1958), *A Comprehensive Dictionary of Psychological and Psychoanalytical Terms*, Longmans, Green & Co., New York

Epictète (1964), *Entretiens*, in *Les Stoiciens*, La Pléiade

Eraly, A. (2000), *L'expression et la représentation – Une théorie sociale de la communication*, Logiques Sociales, L'Harmattan

Erikson, E.H. (1950, 1963), *Childhood and Society*, W.W. Norton and Co., New York (French trans. *Enfance et Société*, Delachaux et Niestlé, Paris, 1982)

Erskine, R. (1995), Shame and self-righteousness, *The British Gestalt Journal*, 2, 107–119

Fairbairn, W.R.D. (1952), *Etudes psychanalytiques de la personnalité*, Ed. du Monde Interne, Paris, 1998

Ferro, A. and Basile, R. (2009), *The Analytical Field: A Clinical Concept*, Karnac Books, London (French trans. *Le champ analytique, un concept clinique*, Ithaque, Montreuil sous Bois, 2015)

Fink, E. (1952), L'analyse intentionnelle et le problème de la pensée speculative. In *Problèmes actuels de la phénoménologie*, Desclée de Brouwer, Paris

Fonagy, I. (1982), *Situation et signification*, John Benjamins, Amsterdam/Philadelphia

Formel, M. and Quéré, L. (eds) (1999), *La logique des situations, Nouveaux ragrards sur l'écologie des activités sociales*, Editions de l'Ecole des Hautes Etudes en Sciences Sociales, Paris

Foucault, M. (1972), Les intellectuels et le pouvoir entretien avec G. Deleuze, *L'arc*, no. 49 (republished in M. Foucault, *Dits et Ecrits I, 1954–1976*, Quarto-Gallimard, Paris, 2001)

Foucault, M. (1977), *Dits et écrits*, Vol II, Quarto-Gallimard, Paris, 2001

Francesetti, G. (2015), From Individual Symptoms to Psychopathological Fields: Towards a Field Perspective in Clinical Human Suffering, *British Gestalt Journal*, vol. 24, no. 1

Francesetti, G., Gecele, M. and Roubal, J. (eds) (2013), *Gestalt Therapy in Clinical Practice: From Psychopathology to the Aesthetics of Contact*, Franco-Angeli, Milan (French trans. *Psychopathologie en Gestalt-thérapie*, L'exprimerie, Bordeaux, 2013)

Freud, S. (1894), *The Neuro-Psychoses of Defence. Standard Edition of the Complete Works of Sigmund Freud* (henceforth SE), 24 vols, Hogarth Press and Institute of Psychoanalysis, London, 1953–74, pp. 43–61 (French trans. Nouvelles remarques sur les névropsychoses-de-défense, in *Œuvres complètes*, III, PUF, Paris, 1989, pp. 120–146)

Freud, S. (1896), Nouvelles remarques sur les névropsychoses de défense (French trans. in *Oeuvres Complètes*, III, Paris, PUF, 1989, pp 130–146)

Freud, S. (1900), *L'interprétation des rêves*, in *Oeuvres complètes*, vol. IV, PUF, Paris, 2003

Freud S. (1905), *Trois essais sur la vie sexuelle*, in *Œuvres complètes*, t. VI, trad. franç. PUF, Paris, 2006

Freud, S. (1905a), *Fragment d'une analyse d'hystérie (Dora)*. In *Cinq psychanalyses*, trans. from German, PUF, Paris, 1954, pp. 1–91

Freud, S. (1905b), *Three Essays on the Theory of Sexuality*, SE vol. 7, pp. 125–145 (French trans. Trois essais sur la théorie sexuelle, in *Œuvres complètes*, VI, Paris, PUF, Paris, 2006, pp. 59–182)

Freud, S. (1912), Conseils au médecin dans le traitement psychanalytique. In *Oeuvres complètes*, vol. XI, PUF, Paris, 1998 (*Recommendations to Physicians Practising Psycho-analysis*)

Freud, S. (1923, 1960) The Ego and the Id. In J. Strachey (ed.) *The Complete Psychological Works of Sigmund Freud*, W.W. Norton, London (French trans. Le moi et le ça, in *Œuvres complètes*, vol. XVI, PUF, Paris, 1991)

Freud, S. (1929), *Civilization and its Discontents*, SE vol. 21, pp. 59–145 (French trans. Le Malaise dans la Culture, in *Œuvres complètes*, vol. XVIII, PUF, Paris, 1994, pp. 245–334)

Freud, S. (1937), La construction dans l'analyse. In *Résultats, idées, problèmes II*, PUF, Paris, 4th edn, 1995 (Constructions in Analysis, in *Findings, Ideas, Problems*)

Freud, S. (1966), Letter to Oskar Pfister, cited in P. Rieff, *The Triumph of the Therapeutic: Uses of Truth after Freud*, Chatto & Windus, London, p. 107

Frie, R. and Coburn, W.J. (eds) (2011), *Persons in Context: The Challenge of Individuality in Theory and Practice*, Routledge, London

From, I. (1978), Interview. Reprinted in W.L. Smith (ed.) *Gestalt Voices*, Ablex Publishing Corporation, Norwood, NJ, 1992 (French trans. *Les rêves, contact et frontière de contact*, Minibibliothèque L'exprimerie no. 88, 1986)

From, I. and Miller, M.V. (1994), Préface. In F. Perls, R. Hefferline and P. Goodman, *Gestalt-thérapie. Vers une théorie du Self: nouveauté, excitation et croissance.* L'Exprimerie, Bordeaux, 2001 (or: Introduction. In F. Perls, R. Hefferline and P. Goodman, *Gestalt Therapy: Excitement and Growth in the Human Personality.* The Gestalt Journal Press, Highland, NY, 1951; 1992

Fromm-Reichman, F. (1960) *Principes de psychothérapie intensive,* Eres

Fuhr, R. and Gremmler-Fuhr M. (1995), Shame in Teaching/learning situations, *The British Gestalt Journal,* 2, 91–100

Fuhr, R. and Gremmler-Fuhr, M. (1997), Shame as Normal and Sometimes Dysfonctional Experience, *Gestalt Review,* vol. 1, no. 3.

Fuhr, R. and Gremmler-Fuhr, M. (2000), La honte comme expérience normale et existentielle. Quelques considérations philosophiques et pratiques. In Clinique de la honte, *Cahiers de Gestalt-thérapie,* no. 7

Gadamer, H.-G. (1960/1990), *Vérité et méthode – Les grandes lignes d'une herméneutique philosophique* (French trans. Coll. L'Ordre Philosophique, Le Seuil, Paris, 1996)

Gagnon, J. (1999), Prendre forme en relation – Fondements pour une compréhension gestaltiste des pathologies limites, *Cahiers de Gestalt-thérapie,* no. 6, L'exprimerie, Bordeaux

Gens, J.-C. (2009), *L'expérience vive,* CNED, PUF, Paris

Gergen, K.J. (1999), *An Invitation to Social Construction,* Sage, London

Gergen, K.J. (2001) *Le constructionnisme social, une introduction,* Delachaux et Niestlé, Lonay

Gergen, K.J. (2005), *Construire la réalité – un nouvel avenir pour la psychothérapie,* Seuil, Paris

Gibson, J.J. (1979), *The Ecological Approach to Visual Perception,* Boston, Houghton Mifflin (French trans. *Approche écologique de la perception visuelle,* Editions Dehors, 2014)

Glassheim, E. (1973), *The Movement Towards Freedom in Paul Goodman's* The Empire City, University of New Mexico, PhD Language and Literature, Modern (pp. 207–208)

Goffman, E. (1964), "La situation négligée" in *Les moments et leurs hommes,* Paris, Seuil/Minuit 1988

Goffman, E. (1974), *Frame Analysis,* French trans. *Les cadres de l'expérience,* Ed. de Minuit, Paris

Goffman E. (1988), L'ordre social et l'interaction, French trans. in Y. Winkin (ed.) *Les moments et leurs hommes,* Seuil/Minuit, Paris

Goldbeter-Merinfeld, E. (ed.) (1998), Constructivisme et constructionnisme social, *Cahiers Critiques de thérapie familiale et de pratique de réseaux* no. 19, DeBoeck Université, Louvain La Neuve

Goldstein, K. (1939/1995), *The Organism: A Holistic Approach to Biology Derived from Pathological Data in Man,* Zone Books (French trans. *La structure de l'organisme,* Gallimard, Paris, 1951)

Goldstein, K. (1940), *Human Nature in the Light of Psychopathology,* Schocken Books, New York, 1963

Goodman, P. (1947), *Kafka's Prayer,* Hillstone, New York, 1976

Goodman, P. (1972), *Little Prayers and Finite Experience,* Harper & Row, New York

Goodman, P. (1977) *Nature Heals,* ed. T. Stoehr, Free Life editions,

Greenberg, L.S. and Paivio, S.C. (1997), Varieties of Shame Experience in Psychotherapy, *Gestalt Review,* 1 (3), 205–220

Groddeck, G. (1923, 1979), *The Book of the It,* Vision Press, London (French trans. *Au fond de l'homme, cela (Le livre du ça),* Gallimard, Paris, 1963)

Groddeck, G. (1970) *Ça et Moi,* French trans. Gallimard, Paris, 1977

Guattari, F. (1995), *Chaosmosis,* Power Publications, Sydney (*Chaosmose,* Galilée, Paris, 1992)

Hall, C.S. and Lindzey, G. (1957), Organismic Theory. In *Theories of Personality,* John Wiley & Sons, New York, pp. 296–335

Harman, R. (1996), Is There a Future for the Here and Now? *The Gestalt Journal*, XIX, 2 (10), 1–108

Héraclite, (1991), *Les fragments*, Les immémoriaux-Fata Morgana

Hermann, I. (1943), *L'instinct filial*, Denoël, Paris, 1972

Hillman, J. and Ventura, M. (1992), *We've Had a Hundred Years of Psychotherapy, and the World's Getting Worse*, Harper San Francisco (French trans. *Malgré un siècle de pssychothérapie, le monde va de plus en plus mal*, Ulmus Company, London, 1998)

Honneth, A. (1995), *The Struggle for Recognition: The Moral Grammar of Social Conflicts* (English trans. of *Kampf um Anerkennung, 1992*), Polity Press, Cambridge, UK (*La lutte pour la reconnaissance*, Cerf, Paris, 2000)

Horwitz, M. (2007), *Courants et pratiques psy*, Coll. L'univers psychologique, Larousse, Paris

Husserl, E. (1913), *Idées directrices pour une phénoménologie*, French trans. TEL, Gallimard, Paris, 1985

Husserl, E. (1929), *Méditations cartésiennes*, French trans. Paris, Vrin 1969

Hycner R. H. (1991), *Between Person and Person – Toward a Dialogical Psychotherapy*, The Gestalt Journal Press, Highland N.Y.

Hycner R. and Jacobs L. (1995), *The Healing Relationship in Gestalt Therapy*, The Gestalt Journal Press, Highland N.Y.

Hycner, R. and Jacobs, L. (1995), *The Healing Relationship in Gestalt Therapy*, The Gestalt Journal Press, Highland, NY

Jacobs, L. (1995), Shame in the Therapeutic Dialogue, *The British Gestalt Journal*, 2, 86–90 (French trans. *La honte dans le dialogue thérapeutique*, Mini-Bibliothèque de Gestalt-thérapie, IFGT, Bordeaux, 2000)

Jacobs, L. (2000), Honte et défenses contre la honte – Ombres sur le dialogue thérapeutique. In Clinique de la honte, *Cahiers de Gestalt-thérapie*, no. 7, p. 97

Jacobs, L. (2010), *Ethical Inspiration and Complex Experiencing*, Kenotes Panel, AAGT Conference, Philadelphia (unpublished typescript)

James, W. (1890), *The Principles of Psychology*, Vol. I, Dover, New York, 1950

James, W. (1912), *Essais d'empirisme radical*, French trans. Agone, Marseille, 2005

Jankelevitch, V. (1980), *Le Je ne sais quoi et le Presque-rien* (Vol. 1: *La manière et l'occasion*), Le Seuil, Paris

Jaspers, K. (1913), *Psychopathologie générale*, Tchou-Les Introuvables, Paris, 2000

Jimenez, M. (2004), *L'esthétique contemporaine*, Klincksieck, Paris

Joas, H. (1992), *La créativité de l'agir*, Cerf, 1999

Jullien, F. (2013), *De l'intime – Loin du bruyant amour*, Grasset, Paris

Jullien, F. (2016), *Près d'elle – Présence opaque, présence intime*, Galilée, Paris

Jullien, F. (2019), *Pourquoi il ne faut plus dire "je t'aime"* – Dialogue avec N. Truong. Ed. de l'aube

Katz, D. (1944), *Introduction à la psychologie de la forme*, trans. from German, Librairie Marcel Rivière & cie, Paris, 1955

Kaufmann, G. (1989), *The Psychology of Shame*, Springer, New York

Kimura, B. (1992), *Ecrits de psychopathologie phénoménologique*, PUF-Psychiatrie ouverte, Paris

Kirschenbaum, H. (1989), *Carl Rogers: Dialogues: Conversations with Martin Buber, Paul Tillich, B.F.Skinner, Gregory Bateson, Michael Polanski and Others*, Houghton Mifflin, New York

Klee, P. (1956/1964), *Théorie de l'Art moderne*, French trans. Denoël/Gonthier, Paris

Klee, P. (1956/1975), *Théorie de l'Art moderne*, Denoël/Gonthier, Paris

Klepner, P. (1999), Exploring Intimacy: A Gestalt Therapy Approach, *The Gestalt Journal*, vol. XXII, no. 2. Republished in D. Bloom and B. O'Neil (eds) *The New York Institute for Gestalt Therapy in the 21st Century*, Ravenwood Press, Queensland, 2014

Lacan, J. (1975), Le séminaire, Livre I; les écrits techniques de Freud, Seuil, Paris

Laplanche, J. and Pontalis, J.B. (1967), *Vocabulaire de la psychanalyse*, PUF, Paris

Lasch, C. (1979), *The Culture of Narcissism: American Life in an Age of Diminishing Expectations*, W.W. Norton & Company, New York (*La culture du narcissisme*, Paris, Champs-Flammarion, 2006)

Lee, R. and Wheeler, G. (1996), *The Voice of Shame, Silence and Connection in Psychotherapy*, Jossey-Bass, San Francisco

Lekeuche, Ph. (1990), La dimension du contact dans la toxicomanie. In Schotte et al., *Le contact*, Brussels, DeBoeck-Wesmael

Levinas, E. (1991), *Entre nous: Essais sur le penser-à-l'autre*, Grasset, Paris

Lewin, K. (1926/1999), Intention, Will and Need? In M. Gold (ed.) *The Complete Social Scientist: A Kurt Lewin Reader*, APA, Washington, pp. 83–115

Lewin, K. (1935), *A Dynamic Theory of Personality*, McGraw-Hill, New York

Lewin, K. (1936), *Principles of Topological Psychology*, McGraw-Hill Book Company, New York

Lewin, K. (1938), *Resolving Social Conflicts*, American Psychological Association, Washington, DC, 1997

Lewin, K. (1951), *Field Theory in Social Science*, Dorwin Cartwright, Harper, New York

Lewin, K. (1952), *Field Theory in Social Science*, Dorwin Cartwright, Tavistock Publications/Routledge & Kegan Paul, London

Lewis, H. Block (1971), *Shame and Guilt in Neurosis*, International Universities Press, New York

Maldiney, H. (1982), La prise. In *Qu'est ce que l'homme? Hommage à Alphonse de Waelhens*, Publication des Facultés Universitaires Saint Louis, Brussels, pp. 135–157

Maldiney, H. (1985), *Art et existence*, Klincksieck, Paris

Maldiney, H. (1986), De la gestaltung, *Psychologie Médicale*, 18 (9), 1419–1422

Maldiney, H. (1990a), Esthétique et contact. In J. Schotte (ed.) *Le contact*, Bibliothèque de pathoanalyse, Editions Universitaires/DeBoeck Université, Brussels

Maldiney, H. (1990b), La dimension du contact au regard du vivant et de l'existant: De l'esthétique-sensible à l'esthétique artistique. In J. Schotte (ed.) *Le contact*, Bibliothèque de pathoanalyse, Editions Universitaires/DeBoeck Université, Brussels

Maldiney, H. (1991), *Penser l'homme et la folie*, Million, Grenoble

Maldiney, H. (1992), Réflexion et quête du soi. In B. Kimura, *Ecrits de psychopathologie phénoménologique*, PUF-Psychiatrie ouverte, Paris

Maldiney, H. (1993), *L'art, l'éclair de l'être*, Ed. Comp'Act

Maldiney, H. (1994a), Esquisse d'une phénoménologie de l'art. In *L'art au regard de la phénoménologie*, Colloque de l'Ecole des Beaux Arts de Toulouse 1993, Presses Universitaires du Mirail, Toulouse

Maldiney, H. (1994b), *Regard, parole, espace*, L'âge d'homme, Lausanne

Maldiney, H. (1997), *Avénement de l'œuvre*, Théétète, St Maximin

Malraux, A. (1949), *The Psychology of Art*, Pantheon Books, New York (*Ecrits sur l'art*, t.II, La Pléiade, Gallimard, 2004)

Marrow, A. (1977), *The Practical Theorist: The Life and Work of Kurt Lewin*, Teachers College Press, New York (French trans. *Kurt Lewin, sa vie et son œuvre*, ESF, Paris, 1972)

Martin, K. (2016), *Le face à face chez Emmanuel Lévinas*, published by the author

McNamee, S. and Gergen, K.J. (eds) (1992), *Therapy as Social Construction*, Sage, London

Mead, G.H. (1934), *Mind, Self and Society, from a Standpoint of a Social Behaviorist*, University of Chicago Press, Chicago (French trans. *L'esprit, le soi et la société*, PUF, Paris, 1963)

Mead, G.H. (1938), *The Philosophy of Act*, University of Chicago Press (7th edn, 1972)

Merleau-Ponty, M. (1945), *Phénoménologie de la perception*, Gallimard, 1976

Merleau-Ponty, M. (1945/2012), *Phenomenology of Perception*, trans. from French by Donald A. Landès, Routledge, London

Merleau-Ponty, M. (1960–1964), *Signs*, North Western University Press, Evanston (French trans. *Signes*, Gallimard, Paris)

Merleau-Ponty, M. (1964), *Le visible et l'invisible*, Gallimard, Paris

Merleau-Ponty, M. (1969), *La prose du monde*, Tel, Gallimard, Paris

Michaux H. (2004), *Vents et Poussières*. In *Œuvres complètes*, vol. III, la Pléiade, Gallimard, Paris

Miller, M.V. (1995), *L'amour terroriste*, French trans. Coll. Réponses, R. Laffont, Paris, 1996

Miller, M.V. (2000), The Myth of We, *The Gestalt Journal*, vol. XXIII, 1, pp. 7–18. In Miller Michael Vincent (2011), *Teaching a Paranoid to Flirt: The Poetics of Gestalt Therapy*, Gestalt Journal Press, Gouldsboro, pp. 167–180

Miller, M.V. (2002), *La poétique de la Gestalt-thérapie*, L'exprimerie, Bordeaux

Miller, M.V. (2004), Preface to J.-M. Robine, *S'apparaître à l'occasion d'un autre.*

Etudes pour la psychothérapie, L'Exprimerie, Bordeaux (republished in M.V. Miller (2011), *Teaching a Paranoid to Flirt: The Poetics of Gestalt Therapy*, Gestalt Journal Press, Gouldsboro)

Minkowski, E. (1966), *Traité de psychopathologie*, Les empêcheurs de penser en rond, Le Plessis-Robinson, 1999

Montaigne, M. (1588), *Les essais*, CFL, Paris, 1969

Morin, E. (1986), *La Connaissance de la connaissance*, vol. 3, Éditions du Seuil, Paris

Mucchielli, A. (2004), *Dictionnaire des méthodes qualitatives en sciences humaines*, 2nd edn, A. Colin, Paris

Nathanson, D.L. (ed.) (1987), *The Many Faces of Shame*, The Guilford Press, New York

Nietzsche, F. (1882), *Le gai savoir*, French trans. Gallimard, Paris, 1982, § 334

Noël, E. (ed.) (1994), *Les sciences de la forme aujourd'hui*, Points-Sciences, Le Seuil, Paris

Pagès, M. (1977), *Le travail amoureux: Eloge de l'incertitude*, Dunod, Paris

Pagès, M. (1990), *L'analyse dialectique: propositions*. Conférence introductive au Colloque de Spetzès (Grèce). Document interne du Laboratoire de Changement Social, Université Paris VII

Parlett, M. (1991), Reflections on Field Theory, *British Gestalt Journal*, 1 (2), 69–81

Perls, F.S. (1943–1992), *Ego, Hunger and Aggression*, The Gestalt Journal Press, Gouldsboro, Maine (*Le Moi, la Faim et l'Agressivité*, Tchou, Paris, 1978)

Perls, F.S., Hefferline R. and Goodman P. (1951), *Gestalt Therapy, Excitement and Growth in the Human Personality*, Julian Press, New York

Perls F.S. (1969a), *Gestalt Therapy Verbatim* (French trans. *Rêves et Existence en Gestalt-thérapie*, Epi, 1972)

Perls, F.S. (1969b), *In and Out the Garbage Pail*, Real People Press (French trans. *Ma Gestalt-thérapie: Une poubelle-vue-du-dehors-et-du-dedans*, Tchou ed., Paris, 1976)

Perls, F. (1973), *The Gestalt Approach*, Sciences and Behavior Books Inc. (French trans. *Manuel de Gestalt thérapie, La Gestalt: un nouveau regard sur l'homme*, ESF, Paris, 2003)

Perls, F. (2019) *Psychopathology of Awareness: An Unfinished and Unpublished Manuscript with Commentary of Contemporary Gestalt-Therapists*, ed. Jean-Marie Robine and Charles Bowman, L'exprimerie, Bordeaux

Perls, L. (1989), *Vivre à la frontière* (French trans. L'exprimerie, Bordeaux, 2001)

Platon, *Théétète*, in *Oeuvres complètes*, vol. 3, trans. from classical Greek, Garnier, VII, 149a–150c

Polster, E. (1966), A Contemporary Psychotherapy: Theory, Research and Practice, 3, 1. In *Recognitions in Gestalt Therapy*, Funk & Wagnalls, New York, pp. 3–19

Polster, E. and Polster, M. (1973), *Gestalt Therapy Integrated*, New York, Random House

Polster, E. and Polster, M. (1976), Therapy without Resistance: Gestalt Therapy. In Burton Arthur (ed.) *What Makes Behavior Change Possible?* Brunner/Mazel, New York, pp. 259–277

Polster, E. (1985), Escape from the Present, Transition and Storyline. In J. Zieg (ed.) *The Evolution of Psychotherapy*, Brunner & Mazel, New York

Ponge, F. (1971), *La fabrique du pré*, Les sentiers de la création/Skira

Prinzhorn, H. (1922), *Expressions de la folie: Dessins, peintures, sculptures d'asiles*. Traduit de l'allemand, Connaissance de l'inconscient, Gallimard, Paris, 1984 (English trans. *The Art of Insanity: An Analysis of Ten schizophrenic Artists*, Solar Books – Solar Research Archive, 2011)

Quéau, P. (1989), *Metaxu*, Champ Vallon, Seyssel

Rank, O. (1929–31), *Volonté et psychothérapie*, Payot, Paris, 1976

Rank, O. (1932), *Art and Artist*, Agathon Press, New York, 1975 (French trans. *L'art et l'artiste*, Payot, Paris, 1984)

Rey A. (ed.) (1992), *Dictionnaire historique de la langue française*, Dictionnaires le Robert, Paris

Rieff, P. (1966), *The Triumph of the Therapeutic: Uses of Truth After Freud*, Chatto & Windus, London

Riker, J. (2009), The Life of the Soul: An Essay in Ecological Thinking, http://www.psychologyoftheself.com/papers/riker.htm

Rimbaud, A. (1912), Lettres dites du Voyant. In *Œuvres complètes*, G.F. La Pleiade, Paris, vol. 1, 2020

Robine, J.-M. (1984), Une esthétique de la psychothérapie. In *Gestalt-thérapie, La construction du soi*, Ed. L'Harmattan, Paris, 1998

Robine J.-M. (1990a), Le contact, expérience première, Revue *Gestalt*, no. 1, Société Française de Gestalt. Republished in J.-M. Robine (1998), *Gestalt-thérapie, la construction du soi*, L'Harmattan, Paris

Robine. J.-M. (1990b), La névrose de champ, *Bulletin de Liaison de la Société Française de Gestalt*, 21–22, 46–63

Robine, J.-M. (1991), La honte, rupture de confluence. In *Gestalt*, 2, 19–34, Republished in J.-M. Robine (1998), *Gestalt-thérapie, la construction du soi*, L'Harmattan, Paris

Robine, J.-M. (1992), Entretien avec Erving Polster, Revue *Gestalt*, no. 3

Robine, J.-M. (1994), De l'étonnement en psychothérapie. In *Gestalt-thérapie, La construction du soi*, Ed. L'Harmattan, Paris, 1998

Robine, J.-M. (1997a), Anxiété et construction des Gestalt, *Cahiers de Gestalt-thérapie* no. 1 (republished in J.-M. Robine, *Gestalt-thérapie, la construction du soi*, L'Harmattan, Paris, 1998 and in G. Francesetti, M. Gecele and J. Roubal (eds) (2013), *Gestalt Therapy in Clinical Practice: From Psychopathology to the Aesthetics of Contact*, Franco-Angeli, Milan)

Robine, J.-M (1997b), La Gestalt-thérapie va-t'elle oser développer son paradigme post-moderne? *Cahiers de Gestalt-thérapie*, no. 5, pp. 59–84 (English trans. in J.-M. Robine (2011), *On the Occasion of an Other*, Gestalt Journal Press, pp. 29–64)

Robine, J.-M. (1998), *Gestalt-thérapie, la construction du soi*, L'Harmattan, Paris

Robine, J.-M. (2001), "From Field to situation" in J.-M. Robine (ed.) *Contact and Relationship in a Field Perspective*, L'exprimerie, Bordeaux (reprinted in *International Gestalt Journal*, vol. 31, no. 1, 2008)

Robine, J.-M. (2002), L'intentionnalité en chair et en os: Vers une psychopathologie du précontact. *Cahiers de Gestalt-thérapie*, no. 12 (republished in J.-M. Robine (2004), *S'apparaître à l'occasion d'un autre: Etudes pour la psychothérapie*, L'exprimerie, Bordeaux)

Robine, J.-M. (2004), *S'apparaître à l'occasion d'un autre: Etudes pour la psychothérapie*, L'exprimerie, Bordeaux

Robine, J.-M. (2005), Le changement social commence à deux, *Gestalt Journal*, no. 29, December

Robine, J.M. (2006a) Gestalt Therapy as Aesthetics. In J.M. Robine (ed.) *La psychothérapie comme esthétique*, L'exprimerie, Bordeaux

Robine, J.M. (ed.) (2006b) *La psychothérapie comme esthétique*, L'exprimerie, Bordeaux

Robine, J.-M. (2007), Quelle figure dévoiler? *Gestalt*, no. 33, Dec., 25–41

Robine, J.-M. (2008), Le maintenant a-t-il un avenir? In P.-Y. Goriaux (ed.), *Le maintenant*, Minibibliothèque de Gestalt-thérapie, no. 110, IFGT

Robine, J.-M. (2010), Contact: At the Source of Experience, *Cahiers de Gestalt-thérapie*, 1 (25), 97–110

Robine, J.-M. (2011a), Ce que je crois et ce que je crois que je crois, *Cahiers de Gestalt-thérapie*, 29, 61–77 (republished in J.-M. Robine (2012) *Le changement social commence à deux*, L'Exprimerie, Paris, pp. 239–250)

Robine, J.-M. (2011b), *On the Occasion of an Other*, Gestalt Journal Press

Robine, J.-M. (2012), *Le changement social commence à deux*, L'Exprimerie, Paris

Robine J.-M. (2015), L'homme de la situation. In H. Cordier and C. Charlier (eds), *Vers une clinique de la situation*, L'exprimerie, Paris

Robine, J.-M. and Lapeyronnie, B. (1996), La confluence, expérience liée et expérience aliénée, *Cahiers de Gestalt-thérapie* (republished in J.-M. Robine, *Gestalt-thérapie, la construction du soi*, L'Harmattan, Paris 1998)

Robine J.-M., Melnick J., Schack M.-L. and Spinelli E. (2007), Contact and Intrapsychic Perspectives: Gestalt Therapists Reply to Questions from the Editors and from Ernesto Spinelli, *Studies in Gestalt Therapy*, vol. 1, no. 2

Robine, J.-M., Miller, M.V., Yontef, G., Lichtenberg, Ph., Spagnuolo-Lobb, M., Philippson, P. and Frazao, L. (2002), *Contact, an Improvised Panel*. DVD-GT. L'exprimerie, Bordeaux

Rose, G.J. (1980), *The Power of Form: A Psychoanalytic Approach to Aesthetic Form*, International Universities Press, Psychological Issues Monograph 49, Madison, Connecticut (2nd edn 1986)

Rosenberg, M.J. (1960), *Attitude Organization and Change: An Analysis of Consistency Among Attitude Components*, Greenwood Press

Salonia G. (2010), Changements sociaux et malaises psychiques. In G. Francesetti, *Attaques de panique et postmodernité*, L'exprimerie, Bordeaux

Sartre, J.P. (1939), *Sketch for a Theory of the Emotions*, Methuen, London, 1956; Routledge, London, 1994 (*Esquisse d'une théorie des émotions*, Hermann, Paris, 1963)

Sartre, J.P. (1943), *Being and Nothingness*, London, Methuen, 1958 (*L'être et le néant*, Gallimard, Paris)

Sartre, J.-P. (1995), *Carnets de la drôle de guerre*, Gallimard, Paris

Schotte et al. (1990), *Le contact*, DeBoeck-Wesmael, Brussels

Serre, J.-P. (1977), *Linear Representations of Finite Groups*, Springer-Verlag, Berlin

Sheldrake, R. (1985), *Une nouvelle science de la vie*, Er Rocher

Shostrom, E.L. (1965), *Three Approaches to Psychotherapy – Part 1: Gloria with Carl Rogers* [Film], Psychological Films, Orange, CA

Simondon, G. (1964), *L'individu et sa genèse psycho-biologique*, J. Millon, 1995

Siomopoulos, V. (1983), *The Structure of Psychopathological Experience*, Brunner/Mazel, New York

Smuts, J.C. (1927), *Holism and Evolution*, Macmillan and Co., London

Spagnuolo-Lobb, M. and Amendt-Lyon, M. (eds) (2003), *Creative Licence: The Art of Gestalt Therapy*, Springer, New York (French trans. Permis de créer, L'exprimerie, Bordeaux, 2006)

Spagnuolo-Lobb, M. (2013), *The Now-for-Next in Psychotherapy: Gestalt Therapy Recounted in Post-Modern Society*, FrancoAngeli, Milan (French trans. Ed. L'exprimerie)

Staemmler, F.M. (2002), The Here and Now, *British Gestalt Journal*, 11 (1), 21–32

Staemmler, F.M. (2003a), *Cultiver l'incertitude*, trans. from English and German, L'exprimerie, Bordeaux

Staemmler, F.M. (2003b), L'ici et maintenant n'est plus ce qu'il était. In *Cultiver l'incertitude*, L'Exprimerie, Bordeaux

Staemmler, F. (2006a), A Babylonian Confusion: On the Uses and Meanings of the Term 'Field', *British Gestalt Journal*, 15 (2), 64–83

Staemmler, F.M. (2006b), The Willingness to Be Uncertain: Preliminary Thoughts about Interpretation and Understanding in Gestalt Therapy, *International Gestalt Journal*, 29 (2)

Steiner, B. and Moralès, G. (1997), *Le style, structure et symptôme*, L'Harmattan, Paris

Stern, D.B. (2003), *Unformulated experience: From Dissociation to Imagination in Psychoanalysis*, Relational Perspectives Book Series, Psychology Press, New York

Stern, D.B. (2010), *Partners in Thought: Working with Unformulated Experience, Dissociation and Enactment*, Routledge, New York

Stern, D.N. (1985), *Le monde interpersonnel du nourrisson*, PUF, Paris, 1988

Stern, D.N. (2003), *The Present Moment in Psychotherapy and Everyday Life*, Norton, New York (French trans. *Le moment présent en psychothérapie*, Odile Jacob, Paris)

Stoehr, T. (1994) *Here, Now Next: Paul Goodman and the Origins of Gestalt Therapy*, Jossey Bass, San Francisco (French trans. Ici, maintenant et ensuite, L'exprimerie Bordeaux, 2012)

Straus, E. (1935a), *Du sens des sens: Contribution à l'étude des fondements de la psychologie*, trans. from German, Millon, Grenoble, 1989

Straus, E.W. (1935b), *Vom Sinn der Sinne, Ein Beitrag zur Grundlegung der Psychologie*, Springer Verlag, Berlin (French trans. *Du sens des sens*, Millon Ed., Grenoble 1989)

Straus, E. (1966a), *Phenomenological Psychology*, Basic Books, New York

Straus, E.W. (1966b), The sigh. In *Phenomenological Psychology*, Basic Books, NY (French trans. Le soupir, introduction à une philosophie de l'expression, *Le cercle Herméneutique*, April 2003, no.1)

Straus, E.W. and Griffith, R.M. (eds) (1970), *Aisthesis and Aesthetics: The Fourth Lexington Conference on Pure and Applied Phenomenology*, Duquesne University Press, Pittsburgh

Melnick, J., Robine, J.-M. Robine, Schack, M.-L. and Spinelli, E. (2007), *Studies in Gestalt Therapy*, Contact and Intrapsychic Perspectives: Gestalt-therapists Reply to Questions from the Editors and from Ernesto Spinelli. Vol. I, no. 2

Szondi L. (1983), *Introduction à l'analyse du destin*, Pathei Mathos, Nauwelaerts, Louvain/Paris

Tatossian, A. *Pratique psychiatrique et phénoménologie* (version abrégée et provisoire), tapuscrit pour un séminaire du groupe de recherches de phénoménologie psychiatrique de Bordeaux. Non daté (années 70), non publié

Tatossian, A. (1979), *Phénoménologie des psychoses*, Masson, Paris

Todorov, T. (1981), *Mikhaïl Bakhtine: Le principe dialogique*, Le Seuil, Paris

Todorov, T. (1995), *La vie commune*, Le Seuil, Paris

Tomkins, S.S. (1963), *Affect, Imagery, Consciousness, vol. II: The Negative Affects*, Springer, New York, 1992

Toulmin, S.E. (1977), Self-Knowledge and Knowledge of the 'Self'. In *The Self: Psychological and Philosophical Issues*, ed. Theodore Mischel, Basil Blackwell, Oxford

Vansteenwegen, A. (1998), Theories et pratiques post-modernes: lecture critique. In *Cahiers critiques de thérapie familiale et de pratique de réseaux*, De Boeck Université, no. 19 (232)

Vincent, B. (2003), *Présent au Monde: Paul Goodman*, L'exprimerie, Bordeaux

Watzlawick, P. (ed.) (1981), *L'invention de la réalité*, French trans. Le Seuil, Paris, 1988

Watzlawick, P., Weakland, J. and Fisch, R. (1975), *Changements, paradoxes et psychothérapie*, French trans. Ed. du Seuil, Paris

Weiszäcker, V. Von (1933), *Le cycle de la structure (Der Gestaltkreis)*, French trans. Desclée de Brouwer, 1958

Wertheimer, M. (1945, 1959), *Productive Thinking*, Harper, New York

Wheeler, G. (1991), *Gestalt Reconsidered, a New Approach to Contact and Resistance*, Gestalt Institute of Cleveland Press & Gardner Press

Wheeler, G. (1996), Self and shame. In R. Lee and G. Wheeler, *The Voice of Shame, Silence and Connection in Psychotherapy*, Jossey-Bass, San Francisco

Whitaker, C. (1982), *From Psyche to System*, ed. J.R. Neill and D.P. Kniskern, The Guilford Press, New York

Wittgenstein, L. (1921), *Tractatus Logico-Philosophicus* (French trans. Tel-Gallimard, Paris, 2001)

Wittgenstein, L. (1989), Remarques sur la philosophie de la psychologie, 1, Mauvezin, Ed. T.E.R. (§869)

Wollants, G. (2005), Interviewed by Parlett M., Therapy of the Situation, *British Gestalt Journal*, vol. 14, no. 2

Wollants, G. (2008/2012), *Gestalt Therapy, Therapy of the Situation*, Sage, London

Worringer, W. (1911), *Abstration et Einfühlung: Contribution à la psychologie du style*, trans. from German, Klincksieck, Paris, 1978

Wurmser L. (1981), *The Mask of Shame*, The Johns Hopkins University Press, Baltimore

Yalom, I.D. (1985), *The Theory and Practice of Group Psychotherapy*, Basic Books, New York

Yontef, G. (1993), *Awareness, Dialogue & Process: Essays on Gestalt Therapy*, Gestalt Journal Press, Highland

Yontef, G. (2000), Relation et sens de soi dans la formation en Gestalt-thérapie, in Clinique de la honte, *Cahiers de Gestalt-thérapie*, no. 7

Yontef, G. (2021), *Gestalt-thérapie relationnelle*, Vol. 2, *L'attitude dialogale*, French trans. L'exprimerie, St Romain la Virvée

Yontef, G. and Jacobs, L. (2002), Gestalt therapy. In R.J. Corsini and D. Wedding (eds) *Current Psychotherapies*, Wadsworth/Thomson Learning, Belmont, CA, pp. 303–339

Zahm, O. (1994), Felix Guattari et l'art contemporain, Revue *Chimères* no. 23

Zarader, J.-P. (2002), *Le vocabulaire des philosophes*, Vol. IV. Philosophie contemporaine, Ellipses, Paris

Zinker, Joseph (1977), *Creative Process in Gestalt Therapy*, Vintage Books, New York

Zweig, S. (1939), *Impatience du cœur*. In *Romans, nouvelles et récits*, Vol. II, French trans. La Pléiade-Gallimard, Paris, 2013

Index

For Product Safety Concerns and Information please contact our EU
representative GPSR@taylorandfrancis.com
Taylor & Francis Verlag GmbH, Kaufingerstraße 24, 80331 München, Germany

9 781032 849485